Med – Chains
&
Covid-19

Innovative Solutions for Pandemics

-Integrating Pandemic Management-

By

Eyong Ebot

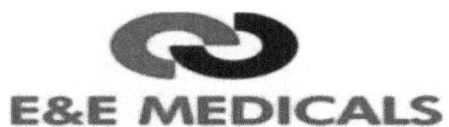

400 Galleria Pkwy Suite 1500
Atlanta, GA 30339

MED - CHAINS© Copyright 2020
by Ebot Eyong

For information about special discounts for bulk
purchases, please contact E&E medicals special
sales at +1-800-305-6069
sales@med-chains.com
sales@eemedicals.com

For more information or to book an event,
contact our speaker bureau at
+1-678-815-9233
or visit our website at
www.med-chains.com www.eemedicals.com

ISBN 978-163732387-8

9 781637   323878

This book is dedicated to my two beautiful daughters, Arielle and Arlyn, and my lovely wife, Cynthia. I also want to dedicate it to my mother, who poured all she had on her children with much resiliency and sacrifice.

TABLE OF CONTENTS

CHAPTER ONE

Introduction

W e are living in odd times, given the current Covid-19 pandemic caused by the spread and contamination of the SARS-CoV-2 virus. A pandemic of this magnitude caused a third of the world's population to become infected with the H1N1 virus a century ago, in 1918, with an estimated fifty million more deaths when compared with mortalities of the first and second world wars. SARS-CoV-2 is an infection that can occur for two days to two weeks without symptoms in the human body and, in some cases, for the entire life of the infection. The COVID-19 pandemic tells the world a human death tale and medical supplies' unavailability to rescue lives.

Bookish innovative ideas are discussed by most news outlets, social media, and medical workers to compensate for the lack of funding. For example, some healthcare workers have worn garbage bags in the absence of hospital gowns. One thing is undeniably real; our healthcare professionals do not have personal protective equipment (PPE) in times of greatest need to protect themselves and provide patients with the best treatment urgently needed.

Forecasts from the Center for Healthcare Metrics and Evaluation (IHME) have shown that there is still a shortage of hospital beds and therapeutics even though adequate protection measures are pursued. It is an inconvenient truth that raises a challenging question: Why does the world experience such medical supply shortages to fight the COVID-19 pandemic? These shortages in most medical facilities and regulatory challenges affect the medical device industry and healthcare systems. Even though a few predicted it, the novel coronavirus pandemic seemed to have started by surprise.

Once exclusive to the Chinese city of Wuhan, the epidemic has gone from a news headline to the talk of every country, media house, community, and professional debate. In a noticeably short period, it is being rated as the fastest disease outbreak in memory. Coronavirus has ushered market failures, where high demand for medical supplies is met with limited supply. It is now a competition for manufacturers and distributors to set new terms and conditions for purchasers. This involves high financial risk payment terms, such as upfront fees, of up to 50%. The balance is due when the goods leave the warehouse.

Over a short period, the emerging economic model has substantial advantages in its offing, particularly for the global market's wealthiest economies. It is exacerbated by the panic buying of people from high-income countries. The disparity has complicated the whole issue and reduced access to affordable and quality-assured medical supplies for countries in the low and middle-income categories. The Zika virus caused defects and neurological issues to thousands of infants. The Ebola virus had a significant impact, particularly in West Africa.

A total of about 45000 cases of Ebola Virus Disease (EVD) and 16000 deaths were reported in Guinea, Liberia, and Sierra Leone. Medical experts suggested that the lack of medical supplies and PPE led to an increased rate of infections. Since then, nothing has significantly changed, putting millions of healthcare workers and patients on thin Covid-19 ice.

Med-Chains is about the interrelations and challenges faced by countries in finding solutions during pandemics. The effects of disruptions within the healthcare system and the activities that lead to shortages in medical supplies, regulatory challenges, government interventions, re-engineering, and geo-economic consequences during a pandemic are relatively connected. The COVID –19 pandemic reveals both the interconnections and cracks in healthcare systems. Med-Chains presents a compelling case for strengthening the global response to pandemics at both international and national levels.

According to credible sources, the economic disruption caused by COVID 19 is in the heights of 35 trillion dollars. The same study estimates show that the next pandemic could be prevented at about 130 billion in the next two years. These estimates are not without error bars, but they provide a perspective from the preliminary findings relating to the urgency to prevent, protect, and respond to such a crisis. In all, the need to strengthen research and development for vaccines and other diagnostics remains imperative.

This book examines advances in solving pandemics, recognize gaps with outstanding healthcare systems' challenges, and encourages all stakeholders to consider such challenges during system improvements. The corresponding chapters focus on building strong response systems, robust detecting mechanisms, and developing healthcare systems with provisions to handle and maintain services invaluable to the public. All these efforts aim at answering a straightforward question: How can we make sure a pandemic of the scale of COVID-19 never happens again?

CHAPTER TWO

COVID –19 Pandemic

The new coronavirus, named SARS-COV-2, is the leading cause of the disease called COVID-19. Discussing the origin of the virus, its spread, comparing it with other diseases caused by coronaviruses, and measuring these diseases' severity is not just relevant but essential. After nearly ten months since the beginning of the pandemic, some people still do not understand its gravity.

What is a coronavirus?

Coronaviruses are a sub-class of the virus family with crown-like spikes on their surface when viewed under the microscope. Many forms of coronaviruses are already in circulation within animals and the human body.

Dromedary camels were associated with the virus causing the Middle East respiratory system (MERS) in 2012. Below is a list of global pandemics in memory.

The first reported case of the novel coronavirus (2019-NCOV) was in December 2019, in Wuhan, the Hubei (China) capi-

Year	Outbreak	First reported	Global death toll	Hosts
1889	Russian flu pandemic	Russia	1,000,000	Avian
1918	Spanish flu pandemic (H1N1)	Spain	50,000,000	Avian
1957	Asian flu pandemic (H2N2)	China	1,100,000	Avian
1967	Marburg virus	Germany/Serbia	475	Fruit bats
1968	Hong Kong flu pandemic (H3N2)	China	1,000,000	Avian — poultry
1976	Ebola	Dem Rep of Congo	218	Fruit bats
1981	HIV/Aids	US	32,000,000	Chimpanzees
2003	Sars (Sars-CoV)	China	774	Bats — civets
2009	Swine flu pandemic (H1N1)	Mexico/US	18,449	Swine
2012	Mers (Mers-CoV)	Saudi Arabia	866	Bats — dromedary camels
2014	Ebola	Guinea	11,300	Fruit bats
2019	Covid-19 pandemic (Sars-Cov-2)	China	1,123,472*	Bats

Selected outbreaks
*As at Oct 22 2020
Sources: WHO;
CDC; ECDC

tal, where approximately 11 million people live. While the emerging virus origin is unknown, most of the new cases were associated with the Huanan seafood wholesale market. Substantial data suggest that this virus is associated with bats, but it remains to be proven.

Coronaviruses affect the respiratory tract, breathing passages, or the airways. Mild symptoms include fever, cough, shortness of breath, and fatigue. Difficulty in breathing is a severe symptom. For MERS (Middle East Respiratory Syndrome) and SARS (Server Acute Respiratory Syndrome), there have been cases of acute illnesses that lead to death.

Currently, it is proven that not all COVID-19 suspected individuals display symptoms of infection. Based on the limited data available, the aging population and those with underlying healthcare conditions suffer the most fatality of the disease.
The virus has infected people from more than 215 countries within a short period; by November29, 2020, it had infected more than 60 million people, and over one and half million deaths were registered.

The death rate surge created a sense of urgency, rushed scientists, biotech entrepreneurs, and engineers to develop coronavirus tracking and distribution models, diagnostic tests, and redesign medical equipment to respond to the global pandemic. The conventional modes of transmitting respiratory viruses occur through droplets or aerosols. Smaller particles join to form aerosols and travel farther distances. Infection by contact involves touching infected objects and contact with infected persons. The disease has been determined to be airborne.

Unless drastic measures are taken to improve efficiency and effectiveness in preventing the virus from spreading, the growing need for better healthcare services has overwhelmed the current healthcare systems. Thus, it is difficult to deal with the current healthcare crisis, let alone mentioning future ones. Apart from the complexities in supply chain management, there are many players and moving parts in the process. Med-Chains contributes to widening our understanding of healthcare systems, medical supplies, personal protective equipment, pharmaceutical, and regulatory challenges as tested and strained by the novel coronavirus pandemic outbreak.

Detecting the Virus

Dr. Anthony Fauci, the leading expert in infectious diseases in the United States of America, said earlier in April that the inability to monitor COVID-19 rapidly and effectively is a failure. Pathogens that emerge and re-emerge require a multidisciplinary approach to achieve their surveillance and detection. These key pathogens' complexity with their diverse tissue tropisms and multiphasic immunological responses goes beyond basic modern medicine. A combined medical history analysis, clinical signs, and physical examination might include a differential diagnosis list, which depends on the approach implemented.

"Laboratory methods are vital to recognize an etiologic agent from testing clinical samples, like blood, nasopharyngeal swab, serum, etc. "

-Wun-Ju Shieh

Today's medical microbial and infectious disease are key factors, which combine with traditional microbiological procedures, conventional immunology research, and modern molecular methods. However, there are logistical and technological problems related to these approaches, and sometimes there is no clinical or pathological connection to the test findings.

Detecting Techniques

Modern pathology techniques involve a morphological pattern recognition method and a traditional wide array of advanced molecular and immunological techniques. These include both traditional methods and new modern methods, which permeate into more spheres of modern medicine. These methods cannot stand alone to detect a virus and complement each other since they all have their advantages and limitations.

A careful evaluation must also be reached to establish their status as a necessary laboratory assay or a diagnostic test to detect the virus using these techniques, saving time, effort, and money.

Polymerase Chain Reaction Assay

PCR amplification has become a common practice in most pathology labs, especially when it comes to the detection of emerging viruses. It allows for high sensitivity, gives rapid and accurate results since molecular identification enhances definitive conclusions. Formalin Fixed Paraffin Embedded (FFPE) samples would allow for effective diagnosis even if the culture were not initially obtained from a biopsy or autopsy when processing the microbial virus.

PCR involves isolating microorganisms' nucleic acids by using gel electrophoresis, restriction endonuclease enzymes, and other nucleic acid hybridization methods. Sometimes when unknown etiological viruses are concerned, degenerate primers are employed in PCR amplification at reduced stringency. This allows for multiple pathogens to be detected simultaneously. It also ensures rapidity, accuracy, and versatility. What has made PCR so accurate and feasible is the usage of 16S Ribosomal RNA (16S rRNA). The pan-eubacterial has a wide range of sequences obtained from the 30S subunit of the prokaryotic ribosomes, which helps in detecting even unknown bacterial or viral specimens.

The availability of this wide range of sequences allows bonding sites for universal PCR primers. Complementary chains can provide a sound analysis of the etiological strains by comparison to the known sequences. However, like other techniques, this technique also has its drawbacks and limitations. The PCR processes are sometimes contaminated. Lax- sterile conditions prevail when the microbial tissues are being processed, increasing the probability of contamination.

The formalin fixation causes fragmentation in the sequence in this technique as well. Often the target gene contains minimal data, no contrast can be made with the pre-existing data, leading to inconclusive results.

Tissue Micro Arrays

This method uses multiplex PCR and other nucleic acid localization methods. It can even be performed on preserved or frozen tissues; however, this gives rise to biosafety concerns. Viral microarrays target 10-100 causative agents and even detect unknown pathogens. Arrays are used to facilitate the PCR process when specific arrays are developed to address a limited number of etiological agents and increase specific genetic targets' frequency. Arrays are also helpful when detecting the gene sequencing of rapidly changing viruses.

Oglio nucleotide microarrays have probes of up to 70 Units; their working is not hindered by RNA viruses changing and evolving. This process is less sensitive than PCR. Other methods are less standardized yet include modern laser capture microdissection (L.C. M), confocal microscopy, proteomics, and in situ polymerase chain reaction assay. These are sparingly being used. They need further research, modification, and optimization to become mainstream methods of detection.

To detect COVID-19, a repeated polymerase chain reaction is used along with a combination of techniques. The nucleic acid and the SARS CoV 2 virus's antigen are detected by a combination of assays for viral testing, which were meticulously decided upon and subsequently authorized. The nucleophiles move into the nasal passages of the affected patient. This became indicative of how the diagnostic process would work. The viral test procedure involves swabs being swept on the patient's nasal passages, larynx, and pharynx. The swabs are then tested for the presence of COVID-19. The diagnosis response is either positive or negative.

A reverse transcriptase-polymerase chain reaction or R.T.-PCR is used on the RNA (ribonucleic acid) of SARS COV 2, which confirms the virus's presence. Tissue samples of severe and fatal cases caused by unknown infectious causative agents are promptly and adequately collected. They are preserved and timely processed. Most are sent to highly specialized centers designed to deal with detecting the virus.

Due to the natural immune response of the body, the strains obtained through the usage of these detection techniques are generally small, and thus multiple clinical samples are required to reach a convincing conclusion about the pathogenesis. The samples must be taken from relevant lesions that undergo histopathological changes. The most important thing is the correlation between different results where the intangibles are possibly controlled. The results and factors include everything from clinical history, laboratory assays, and epidemiology data.

Molecular Mechanism

Molecular pathways are one of the fundamental approaches used to diagnose the infection of COVID-19. Coronavirus key cellular entry depends on protein binding with viral spicules (S) to cellular receptors and S protein priming by host cell proteases. The SARS-CoV-2 virus has been shown to use the pulmonary alveoli-level ACE2 receptor for entry along with the enzyme TMPRSS2 serine protein for the initiation of protein S. Approximately 80% of COVID 19 infections are moderate. Patients with SARS-CoV-2 in convalescents have a neutralizing antibody reaction, which can be observed even 24 weeks after infection and is generally directed toward proteins.

Additionally, experimental SARS vaccines, including recombinant S protein and inactivated virus, induce responses to neutralizing antibodies. However, confirmation of the infectious virus is currently suggesting that neutralizing high antibody responses against SARS may provide a little protection against SARS-CoV-2 infection.

The serological immunological test takes 20-30 minutes to obtain rapid test data. The antibody test results are obtained only a few days after the blood antigens develop. These assessments are not ideal for the detection of active infections in the first stage of the disease.

The test investigates the existence of unique anti-corona-virus (SARS-CoV-2) antibodies, IgG, and IGM, respectively. However, it should be noted that such a simple test does not help early diagnosis because its results are gotten between three to five days after the disease begins. Simply put, the test may be favorable for an asymptomatic person who over three to five days after infection.

Secondly, the NA test gives 20-30 minutes to calculate the viral antigen, like quick influenza testing. These quick tests are rugged more than serological tests, as they help detect new coronavirus infections early and diagnose them early. Currently, an ideal testing method has not been determined.

"That is why I suggest the government appoints one senior minister of capability whose sole task is to step up to the challenge of producing testing capacity, both PCR and antibody. Alongside him or her should be a team that includes businesspeople familiar with industrial production and procurement; and of course, those with the scientific expertise."

- Tony Blair, Former Prime Minister of the United Kingdom.

Tracking and Preventing transmissions

The coronavirus is constantly spreading throughout the world. The virus has a high transmission rate; however, studies have revealed that the patients who test positive for the virus are of two types; asymptotic patients and symptomatic patients. Asymptotic patients are carriers of the virus and test positive for it; however, they do not threaten transmissions. They can be treated at home and do not require isolation. After the infection of the patient is established, they do not affect anyone through contact.

To track the virus, people with travel history, those who come into contact with travelers, those who were living in heavily affected areas, and those exhibiting the typical symptoms (fever, cold, cough, bodily aches) are asked to isolate themselves for fourteen days and are tested over this period. If they test positive, the treatment starts, and if they test negative, they are required to complete their 14-day quarantine/ isolation period. This can be done at home or in government-organized isolation setups.

Canada introduced tracking via phone cameras to ensure people stuck to these regulations. Other countries also introduced house arrest bands, which would beep and signal the relevant departments if the subject moved out of the set perimeters. Since COVID-19is now a pandemic, all countries must notify the National Notifiable Diseases Surveillance System (NNDSS) about the number of patients who test positive and the number of deaths. As such, viruses should be tracked regarding, which area prevents their development or which area has controlled the virus's spread, so prevention, control, and management techniques can be studied and implemented.

Moreover, this data helps monitor the virus's epidemiology and help develop models that depict the virus's trend and frequency. For example, when is it supposed to rise, what areas will it spread into, will there be a dip, and will there be a second or third wave? More so, they also give us data related to patient' progress and their recovery. Which gender is getting more affected, what age group?

Did they have any underlying medical health conditions, which exacerbated the situation? What is the average recovery period? What are the most common drugs that are treating the virus? Does the sample collection method involve incidence, prevalence, hospitalizations, and deaths? These are all questions we continue asking experts.

The data collected is then divided into different categories, multiple pie charts, data tables, frequency graphs are made to depict the data. These visualizations are continuously updated and help the public and scientists.

Identification and Isolation of COVID-19 Cases

- Early isolation and detection of potentially infectious people is a vital first step towards the safety of staff, guests, and workers in workplaces where exposures to COVID 19 can occur.

- Isolate persons suspected of getting COVID 19 instantly, as far as possible. Infectious people for example, travel to isolation rooms. If air safety is not jeopardized, potentially infective people are moved on aircraft to crew and passengers' seats.

- Take measures to reduce the transmission of contagious respiratory secretions, including supplying them with a face mask. After isolation, depending on the kind of workplace isolated persons should quickly exit the workplace. Depending on their condition's seriousness, they may be ready to return to their home or seek help; however, some people may need emergency health care services for themselves.

- In healthcare environments, isolate patients suspected of COVID 19 separately to avoid further spread, including screening, triages, and treatment facilities, from all patients with confirmed cases of the virus.

  I. Limit workers in isolation areas such as a patient's kitchen with COVID 19 suspected or even confirmation.

II.   Protect the employees by using more engineering and EPIs, safety work, and management controls in close contact with the deceased individual.

III.   Sick employees are expected to leave the workplace fast. Based on the nature of the isolated employee's disease, he or she may be ready to return or even seek medical attention for herself, although certain people may need emergency medication.

The Center for disease control(CDC) in the United States describes close contact within 6 feet, with no prescribed PPE, of an infected individual. Near contact also involves cases in which contact with infectious secretions happens instantly without the use of advisable PPE. Near communication does not necessarily involve short encounters, such as bypassing someone.

Environmental Decontamination and Cleaning

If people affect a surface or maybe substance infected with SARS-CoV-2, they may be exposed to the disease. According to the CDC, the National Health Institutes, and other research collaborators, SARS-CoV-2 can live for 2 to 3 days on some surfs, such as stainless steel and plastic steel. However, since the communicability of SARS-CoV-2 from polluted surfaces and environmental items is not well known, employers should carefully consider whether work areas occupied by those suspected of the disease may be contaminated and whether they should be decontaminated in response.

Does the CDC provide environmental purification and disinfection guidance for different types of workplaces, including health services and guidelines on prevention of infections as part of CDC treatment services such as postmortem employers in COVID 19 pandemic workplaces and other facilities?

The use of SARS-CoV-2 approved disinfectants of the EPA should be employers who need to clean and disinfect areas potentially polluted with SARS-CoV-2. Routines and disinfection methods are ideal for SARS-CoV-2, including inpatient treatment areas in aerobically-producing medications, e.g., using water and purifiers to pre-clean surfaces before using an EPA registered disinfectant frequently contaminated surfaces or objects, for sufficient contact times as specified on the product label.

COVID-19 Tracking Apps

The production of vaccines could sometimes take many months. Hence, one of the methods to reduce the virus's spread depends on how infected individuals could be tracked and isolated using contact-tracing apps. Such endeavors have been successful in China and South Korea. The Smartphone app tracks the tested individuals and notifies others who come close to someone identi-fied with the virus. Such innovative moves encourage individuals to distance themselves from contaminated patients in both public and private areas.

"As the industry moves to accelerate interventions for the treat-ment and prevention of COVID-19, the stakes are incredibly high," Carolyn Magill, CEO of Aetion, said in a statement. "Our offerings use Health Verity's comprehensive, real-time data to obtain decision-ready insights that can help meet the need for ac-celerated approvals and access, while maintaining our high bar for evidence to support critical safety and effectiveness determinations."

Testing Challenges

The testing results obtained from millions of individuals for COVID – 19 show inaccurate positive and negative results. The R.T.- PCR (reverse transcriptase-polymerase chain reaction) varies for individuals from the symptom onset. The false-negative test for the virus is now a long-term problem that has overshadowed test availability concerns. Inaccurate results of the diagnostic test are un-dermining all other efforts to contain the pandemic. Both false pos-itive and false negative results are consequential. The Food and

Drug Administration (FDA) has approved commercial test devices, but the approved machines' sensitivity differs.

Companies' clinical tests, which are approved through the EUA process could involve a mixture of both symptomatic and asymptomatic individuals whose sensitivity is doubtful because some swabs might not trap the infected material. Testing device manufacturers are challenged to design devices with integrated reference standards for SARS-COV-2 measurements. Such Standards could solve sensitivity issues related to asymptomatic individuals. We do not currently have an adequate assessment of asymptomatic individuals.

Testing shortages

Controlling transmissions of COVID-19 pandemic requires adequate testing with efforts laying on the availability of the diagnostic supplies. Shortages of diagnostic supplies have been a problem, particularly the unavailability of testing reagents. The molecular assay technology is mostly applied on a much larger scale because it identifies the genetic material, which signals the present infection. The other immunoassays identify antigens or antibodies.

The testing process constraints lie on five identified issues: logistics, sample collection, data management, execution, and testability. To mitigate these shortages observed, it would be essential to look at both short and long-term measures. These measures require a degree of investment and a change in supply and demand procedures that lead to faster results.

Mitigating Measures

Establishing new laboratory, testing, and visibility capacities facilitate testing capabilities and streaming data to the centers on time are key measures. Such measures will help to manage the results and provide information on the inventory level of available reagents. The data obtained will be used by government agencies to plan to prevent shortages.

Optimizing the laboratories' workflow and training qualified personnel is key to adequate results. Laboratories experts complain of the lack of understanding involved in distinguishing between close and open systems. Furthermore, the equipment necessary to provide full task capabilities is lacking. The shortage of testing kids invites bottlenecks, but open systems that run results through more comprehensive ranges significantly impact the testing capacity.

"The BinaxNOW rapid antigen test and complementary mobile app called NAVICA are life-changing technologies that will attack the pandemic on several critical fronts – speed, simplicity, affordability, access, and accuracy. It will help us be more confident as we navigate work, school, and life."

- Robert Ford, President and

CEO of Abbott Laboratories

Approving the laboratory system has become a problem. Establishing information centers, which act as a central repository on kits performances and the identified components, could help speed the validation process of the required test data or ranges from the suppliers and provide suitable bases for measuring manufacturing capacity.

At-Home Coronavirus Test

In a long-awaited development, the Food and Drug Administration approved the first prescription at-home coronavirus test. Lucira Health has developed a test that can be used for at least 14 years of age. The procedure involves swabbing the inside of the nose, putting the swab into a test device. The results could be obtained with a half hour.

"While COVID-19 diagnostic tests have been authorized for at-home collection, this is the first that can be fully self-administered and provide results at home," FDA Commissioner Stephen Hahn said.

A second at-home test using a different technological method should be provided to validate the findings to minimize false positives.

Personal Protective Equipment (PPE)
&
Supplier Relationship Management
(SRM)

Personal Protective Equipment are protective clothing, gloves, helmets, face shields, surgical masks, goggles, respirators, and other equipment designed to safeguard one from injury or prevent one from exposure to infectious disease. PPE is often used in healthcare facilities like hospitals, clinical laboratories, food production, and service facilities. Effective use of PPE includes the appropriate removal and discarding of contaminated equipment to avoid exposing both the user and other individuals.

Medical Supplies for Front-liners

The new coronavirus is different. With this virus, we have an invisible and deadly enemy, and the task is more complicated than other diseases.

Our understanding of disease transmission and treatment is much ahead than in the nineteenth century. Still, this new coronavirus has shown the limits of our ability to deal with significant disease outbreaks. Advice for protection is obvious:

- Wash hands thoroughly and often isolate yourself if you feel uncomfortable.
- Maintain social distance
- Avoid crowded areas and public places.

During the Ebola outbreak, the World Health Organization (WHO) estimated that healthcare workers were 21 to 32 times more possibly infected by Ebola than others in the general adult population. In West Africa, over 350 health workers died in the battle against Ebola. The World Healthcare Organization has mentioned that an increasing disruption in personal protective equipment global supply is endangering lives.

Government and private companies need to act quickly in amending export restrictions, stop speculation and hoarding. We cannot terminate COVID-19 without first protecting healthcare workers. PPE prices have risen significantly since the beginning of the COVID-19 outbreak. Based on WHO models, the response of COVID-19 needs an estimated 79 million medical masks every month. The market for safety glasses has risen to around 109 million.

WHO issued a statement calling on governments to provide incentives for industries to increase production and reduce restrictions on the export and distribution of medical supplies related to the pandemic.

Doctors, nurses, caregivers, and paramedics face unprecedented workloads in congested health facilities with no end in sight. Their work is stressful and terrifying not only because the effects of the virus are poorly understood but also because they are unsecured, overworked, and vulnerable to infection in most situations.

The risk involved for doctors, nurses, and others at the frontline is troubling.

"During the COVID-19 pandemic, we remain committed to helping these individuals who are at the greatest risk, through product donations, redistribution efforts for protective items, virtual volunteer opportunities, and support and donations for frontline and healthcare workers."

- David Heath, Founder of Bombas

Italy has seen nothing less than 30 doctors die of coronavirus. Spain reported that about 3,900 health workers had been infected. In the United States of America, more than 1900 frontline workers have died from the disease. We must do everything in our ability to support health professionals who directly step into the path of COVID-19 to help those affected and stop the spread despite their well-known fears.

"As Churchill said during World War II, never have so many relied on the efforts of so few, there are currently 3 million registered nurses in the U.S., the highest percentage of healthcare workers. You've seen the images of them working overtime in crowded hospitals, you've heard the emotional stories: Nurses giving dying patients their cell phones so they can say goodbye to their loved ones."

- Chris Cuomo, CNN prime time

A recent survey of National Nurses United (NNU) found that only 30% believed that their healthcare organization had sufficient PPE to respond to COVID-19. In some France and Italian areas, hospitals have no masks; doctors are forced to examine and treat COVID-19 patients without adequate protection.

Health facilities need support staff for cleaning light switches, handrails, countertops, and doorknobs frequently using disinfectants. Such measures provide much-needed reassurance as well as less stress to caregivers in protecting the public. Just like soldiers, health workers also face significant mental stress. It is often forgotten that they feel the grief of loss when their patients die from the virus.

They also have families; of course, they are afraid that the virus will reach loved ones if exposed. The heroism, dedication, and selflessness of medical staff give people a level of assurance that the virus can be overcome. These health care soldiers need the support required to carry out their duties, stay alive, and be safe.

"Please hold onto your families tight. Please be safe, don't give up hope. We're going to get through this, I promise. God bless you!"

-Beyoncé Knowles, American singer

Supplier Relationship Management (SRM)

The systemic change of modern society (e.g., mobility, aging of the population) and the rising dynamics of the market forces companies to decrease costs and enhance services. Supplier Relationship Management is an approach that structurally handles the relationships of a company with its suppliers. These partnerships lead to cost savings and enhance the quality of service during the pandemics.

During a crisis, the buyer and supplier's trust are low, and the communications were conflicting. In effect, SRM has not received much interest in healthcare practice, unlike other electronics or the car industry. Adopting electronic services reduces planning and submitting requests for paper bills and removes costly manual entry errors. Electronic orders are executed only by 39 percent of German hospitals and 36 percent through electronic invoices. In contrast to the airline market, 85% of companies actively use e-commerce in their daily operations. The handling, sorting, and procurement orders account for 33 to 40% of hospital supply costs. It should be less than 11 percent in a competitive industry.

Hospital procurement departments are also helping to improve revenue and the acquisition of expertise. Thus, the supplier's position previously regarded as an opponent (for example, in price negotiations) is transformed into an enterprise partner, which adds value to the hospital. Suddenly, more outstanding teamwork, collaboration, and communication in healthcare activities should be expected.

Services for SRM

Because SRM consists of both social and technical components, a holistic approach is required to improve healthcare systems. The process framework for this system consists of general business and management processes for handling relationships with suppliers.

The framework includes the following areas:

Governance: We must develop and execute the sourcing, monitoring, and controlling strategy. We need to define goals and working methods and respond to changes by changing plans in case of disruptions.

Strategic Sourcing: Initiating, negotiating, and stabilizing supplier relationship and operational purchasing, i.e., determining the required goods, ordering the requested goods, and handling the trade dynamics that challenge effective performance is what our hospitals need in the future. The framework includes support models that are vital for professional and social networks.

Human Resources: Recruiting new professionals, developing current staff, evaluating current staff capacities and performance, and rewarding satisfactory performance is vital areas to be considered.

Infrastructure and IT Services: Documentation of business architecture, alignment of IT capabilities, material flows, optimization of information, and infrastructure renewal with business needs. SRM Software services should be used to process and distribute information within and among the organizations to support the defined processes' completion.

Customer Relationship Management (CRM)

There are technical and social opportunities that assist hospitals in the structured management of customer relations. The outbreak of COVID-19 is showing shortages of the supply chain. Other COVID-19 logistic issues of the medical supply and drug supply chains are predicted as the epidemic evolves. To recognize and address interruptions to the supply chain managers, health facilities must study and optimize their supply chain management tools. Delays in the supply chain call for essential monitoring of established inventory. Many automated systems may be used to track goods from the end of production to the actual patient department.

Many of these programs should adequately handle all medical supplies in a healthcare facility. Real-time analysis provides site leaders with an awareness of inventory levels and other capacities, such as precocious product loss detection. In installations without an integrated inventory management system, care should only be taken to track initial monitoring of a small number of critical medical supplies, which may be insufficient to understand the institutional needs.

Inventory management without automatic monitoring is possible for small companies. A continuous manual process for extremely critical products should determine product usability and specifications in an updated fashion. Continuous supplies like ventilators are required to support respiratory diseases, medicines for respiratory disorders, such as antimicrobials, and bronchodilators, should be monitored.

Purchase Management

If suppliers and distributors have commodity needs they cannot fulfill, the requested products are always distributed in fractions to medical facilities based on previous procurement. Health institutions should recognize the need for essential items to be purchased in the organization. In this way, various non-permitted uses, like vital services or even personal usage, maybe stopped from ordering essential items in shortcomings.

Orders should be preferably made using a centralized, automated mechanism to position order controls on a medical product to enable the procurement of goods from high-priority working units. Thus, purchasing units' approval shall be minimized. If automated procurement control is not feasible, manual processes should prioritize essential goods with vendors, suppliers, and healthcare coalitions.

In the case of disruptions to the supply chain, medical centers should work closely with their vendors and suppliers to develop a shared understanding of the facility requirements, the extent of the disruption, and the anticipated duration. Hospitals need to work on memorandums to understand and share processes in a scarcity period with local and regional health partners. If not, it will exacerbate the situation as local distributors are also under pressure for emergency facilities.

When disturbances to the supply chains are overcome, essential inventories of goods can be replenished with fractional intermediate maintenance. For example, the 5-year shelf life for a product will help stabilize the product supply chain and increase manufacturing potential. Although it is widely thought, by re-stocking at 20 percent per year, or by 10 percent increases, this similar approach can also allow individual healthcare providers to represent their usage and needs more accurately during a crisis. An inventory and routine healthcare system must have shelf-life data to prevent needless waste.

Healthcare institutions should set up an external supply chain risk program or include this in an existing program to make better institutional supply chain decisions, to help institutions better predict future disruptions in supply chains. This involves knowledge of the manufacture of essential goods, including the raw material source. It encompasses a wide range of potential threats, including meteorological, geopolitical, and epidemiological hazards. A detailed review may help integrate these external threats with the vulnerabilities of the supply chain.

An organization may provide helpful information on imminent deficiencies leading to detection and early implementation of substitute products or conservation strategies.

Increase Demand for Medical Devices

Although many companies have unfortunately seen declining demand, such as orthopedics, after elective surgery cancellation and contact lens manufacturers as opticians' closings for non-essential treatments, many companies have adapted their activities to fight COVID-19. Some test equipment manufacturers have redesigned their factories to focus on the development of detection devices for the virus. Also, surgical equipment manufacturers have seen an increase in demand as the National Health Service (NHS) in the UK seeks to ensure adequate supplies.

Even with the demand for products, the continuity of the company is not without challenges. Medical device manufacturing companies continue facing shortages in raw materials and staffing during this critical period. Companies generally purchase raw materials from new suppliers. However, this takes plenty of time, and some find it challenging to find suppliers who meet adequate quality and production standards. Most companies have directed all non-essential workers to work from home and attended video conferencing instead of meetings, but workers in the manufacturing sector cannot work from home.

Firms have been showing their innovation in splitting their shifts, reducing workforce numbers to allow shifts capacity to maintain a six feet distance between workers. Companies should innovate their supply chains. For example, Hope Technologies, a British bicycle parts manufacturers, has redefined the production process and equipment to build parts by automation.

Share Production Knowledge

We have already seen companies changing to voluntary production of PPE to meet excessive demand. For example, a French company, LVMH, is a perfume factory that has decided to produce hand sanitizer and gloves. Puig's fragrance and fashion company offered one of its production shifts to producing hydroalcoholic and disinfecting solutions in Spain. In Italy, pharmaceutical company Menarini has converted its production facility to produce and donate disinfectant gel.

In the UK, distillery companies now produce hand sanitizer, and French Pernod Ricard confirmed that it is supplying 96% distilled alcohol to manufacturers of disinfectant gel in the UK, France, Ireland, and Sweden. There are specific, practical limitations to manufacturing companies' capacity to produce technically complicated and highly regulated products. Meeting the stringent requirements of manufacturing medical devices requires existing medical device manufacturers to be willing to provide new entrants with significant amounts of information, training, and knowledge of new companies before their operations.

Design information, software, machining templates, quality assurance, and other protocols for acceptable manufacturing practices in the medical device industry should be provided to speed up production. Such data are generally considered confidential business secrets, and there are no mandatory licenses or exceptions from government use for trade secrets. Governments may need to rely on the ability to claim goods, as noted above, or create new laws to recover such materials or on a consensual approach to address such short outcomings during pandemics.

Regulatory challenges with Startups

Medical equipment such as ventilators is subject to rigorous regulatory control and long manufacturing approval processes for safety reasons. Considering the urgency of the present global situation, the fastest solution for increasing production capacity is that new manufacturers rely on existing, approved production procedures, quality assurance programs, and conformity certificates from existing medical device manufacturers.

These goals could be achieved through standard manufacturing contracts between an authorized Original Equipment Manufacturer (OEM) of medical equipment and the new manufacturer. Such production schemes allow the production of 'clone' devices in another factory under the quality assurance systems and certificates of conformity of an existing OEM, thereby adding production capacity as quickly and safely as possible.

An extra measure to propel the speed of marketing medical devices and protective equipment occurs when governments relax enforcement and regulatory approvals, but safety must not be compromised. For instance, the EU/EEA market commission recommendation / 2020/403 of March 2020 on the procedures for conformity assessment and market surveillance under the COVID-19 threat recognizes that it is imperative to make sure that the medical devices and protective equipment are safe for end-users.

CHAPTER FOUR

Medical Supplies
&
Geo-economic Challenges

With the development and rapid advancement of technologies, the medical devices industry is probably the fastest growing industry. However, many countries have little access to quality devices and resources that are tailored to epidemiological needs. These conditions relate more to developing countries, where health technology and reliable tests are uncommon, and there are few regulatory controls to avoid the importation or use of modern medical equipment. It threatens undesirable business influences and jeopardizes the lives of patients.

A supply chain from Asia, Europe, and the United States have setbacks considering the global restrictions and stringent export conditions. The transportation of millions of medical equipment and doses of drugs within untested and complex chains makes it even more difficult for supplies to reach appropriate destinations. The unprecedented supply volumes seem challenging to speed transfers from development to manufacture and distribution.

Acute insufficiencies of personal protective equipment have been one disappointing aspect of the COVID-19 catastrophe. One possible reason for the lack of emergency stockpile in sufficient quantities is the depletion of the stockpile from other outbreaks, which happened a few years ago and was never replenished. There were not enough stockpiles to 'fight' the COVID-19 pandemic in many countries.

First, only a few entrepreneurs understand the marketing dynamics of medical kits. When there is a crisis, people complain about "price gouging," which gives politicians the impetus to enforce certain price limits for these items. In contrast, they encourage sellers to make these items available even at a higher competitive market price. Another reason for the shortages is based on the law of supply and demand. China was producing half of the world's face masks before the coronavirus outbreak. Hence, they started hoarding what remained after the virus took off in Wuhan, China.

The problems will only increase as more countries are hoarding what is available. Even Germany banned the export of PPE. Some public health officials shamefully went to the extent of putting out information in the media that face masks cannot protect people from being infected.

Fortunately, this media campaign backfired. The public found scientific proof that the information was not correct, but they also discovered that the face mask saves many lives.

Government Negligence

Before this current pandemic, many governments never had programs or structures that could respond to a massive pandemic. One of the problems they identified was "insufficient personal protective equipment," Besides, some countries could not meet PPE demands to combat such a massive outbreak. Thus, these countries sought help from other governments, but their requests and submissions were met with "confusion" and "bureaucratic chaos."

The failure to store up PPE supplies as strategic stockpiles or ensure an increase in capacity to boost production during an emergency well before the coronavirus pandemic remains pathetic. According to experts and advocates, many governments typically underfund disease outbreak preparedness and public health programs. Though the USA strategic national stockpile still has about 12 million N95 respirators and 20 million surgical masks. It can only meet one percent of the country's needs in a full-blown pandemic.

Doctors and nurses used homemade equipment, trash bags, and bandanas in place for actual protective gear.

Other reasons for the shortage of personal protective equipment, which may not be as significant as previously mentioned, are road-blocks and quarantine measures constraining medical supplies transportation.

Precarious Supply Chain Challenges

In most economies, hospitals are one of the most resource-dependent institutions. Almost nothing is produced, while a continuous supply from external sources is consumed. Research has shown that inventories constitute an average of 15% of overall hospital expenditures but can rise to 40% during pandemics.

The streamlined, time-conscious approach does not allow for storage. For example, with a COVID-19 pandemic, shortages could be observed on almost all supplies needed in most facilities. Many "non-urgent" medical services, which were reduced or stopped (like Surgeries and special medical expert consultations),can no more be postponed.

What can be done if these procedures can no longer be delayed? Are the hospitals fitted with personal safety systems, operating equipment, and hospital beds? What about the sedatives, pain killers, and anesthesia? In the coming months, there are likely to be other prescription shortages.

"We witnessed runson hydroxychloroquine after President Trump touted the drug as an unproven treatment for COVID-19,

making it hard to find for patients who use it regularly for lupus and rheumatoid arthritis. "

– Eugene Scheller

In addition to the increase in demand, supply shortages have plagued the pharmaceutical industry, as existing manufacturing operations are disrupted globally. After Hurricane Maria, companies with factories in Puerto Rico encountered major disorders and lost their full production potential for months because the medical device industry pharmaceutical industry faced similar problems.

Now we must all predict the challenges associated with the tiered medical supply chain so that the ongoing waves of coronavirus can be combated while meeting our people's everyday needs.

To coordinate supply chains, the FEMA Supply Chain Stabilization Task Force, The White House Coronavirus Task Force, and other federal and state agencies can not only concentrate on immediate needs but have an infrastructure ready for the threats that lie in the future. Health organizations need better coordination and exposure in chains providing medical equipment and other supplies. To develop plans to respond to institutional and community needs within the coming months, they need to reinforce relations with manufacturers, distributors, and group procurement organizations (GPOs). Supply chain administrators and intermediaries need their stocks, contingencies, and risk management strategies to be transparent.

There is also the main feature for "talk users," who rent equipment for exceptional demand times like hospital fans. Surprisingly, nothing has been said about these organizations. We must also foresee what equipment, pharmaceuticals, and human resources are needed to address our most urgent needs in the coming years, if not months. The federal governments should relax specific rules, such as widening the practice to assist critical areas in the private sector during pandemics. Health care providers must maintain partnerships, facilitate engagement, and fast recovery of required skills with retiring and redundant workers.

Our healthcare system cannot continue to function in the same way, even with a coronavirus cure. The risk of considering supply chains only in terms of cost savings has been revealed in this crisis. The federal government should promote public health facilities and reserves for high-risk and low-risk risks commodities. Health professionals and executives need more preparation to make supply chain decisions that influence their clinical perspectives.

Although there has been no precedent in the scale of the COVID-19 pandemic, we are facing an imminent lack of vital resources because most health care facilities have not been encouraged to integrate emergency structures to sustain pandemics. We will need to foresee what materials and human resources are needed to address our most pressing needs in the coming years. As COVID-19 continues to spread like wildfire, manufacturers of medical devices typically have design specifications to comply with regulations. Although the regulatory criteria for critical PPE are considerable, the conditions currently in place are not acceptable.

The design specifications that annoy manufacturers need to be versatile. There are now several variations of prototypes instead of a single, clinically diligent PPE prototype. Tom McNulty of Autodesk and Bill Schonger of MakeIt Labor have already set an example of this model.

They presented an overview of how they can efficiently handle group efforts by coordinating many suppliers, creating products that are hard to get, disseminating clinical input, and quickly delivering clinically-controlled PPE.

Geo - Economic Challenges

As the incidence of COVID-19 rises in the USA and around the world, the possible effect of the pandemic on the medical device industry is also being challenged. Presently, predictions of an adverse effect on the US healthcare system and medical devices' distribution becomes more apparent.

Healthcare systems and medical device distributors' efficiency are performance measures intended to provide medical device manufacturers with information about a pandemic in real-time. Although COVID-19 in Mainland China affects tens of thousands of lives, the effect on international supply chains grows daily. China is a major supplier of essential components such as printed circuit boards and complex medical devices in the medical device industry. The effects of a shuttered factory will be felt in the short and long term.

Today, China is the fourth largest medical technology provider in the United States. The Food and Drug Administration (FDA) approved more than 60 percent of controlled products from China. More than $800 million have been invested in China's medical technology industry in the last 15 years by US firms. These investments concentrate on the development of new plants or the expansion of existing plants. Consequently, China's supply chain has been the biggest driver in the US medical device industry.

The flipping nature of this dependency has been demonstrated by recent developments in trade wars and COVID-19. In China, manufacturers of both parts and finished equipment struggle to keep their factories open. The amount of equipment produced has reportedly decreased. The transportation of such equipment is postponed because flights are canceled to/from affected areas. In addition, goods exported from China or rejected once they reach their destination. US companies should perceive this as more than just China's problem.

These phenomena and related problems are starting to appear in many regions outside China. For example, Europe, Africa, and South America face shortages in both the development and availability of medical equipment. The potential for supply chain impacts, irrespective of which country the output takes place, increases as countries are affected. Therefore, to the least, a temporal open border cooperation policy is necessary during such a period.

National lockdowns, shut-down airspaces, and closed borders all go together to prove that Covid-19 has resulted in an unexpected disruption in many economies. In a specific sense, the erection of such barriers has placed a significant strain on the global supply chain performance. Many commercial airlines temporarily repurpose their civilian aircraft to supply the countries affected by COVID 19 with Medical supplies. During this time, the short, medium, and long-term dynamics in pharmaceutical supply chains have proved harder than in recent ones.

Furthermore, a significant reorganization of supply chains outside China and India may result from short-term disruptions in the pharmaceutical sector. It can lead to long-term advantages for local companies and other emerging markets, experts claim. This is especially critical for markets that are responsible for the so-called yellow slice of the global economy.

Specifically, if the pharma supply chains are realigned, there are potential benefits to countries with large internal markets. Interruptions have prevailed in the supply of pharmaceuticals and medical supplies, but the latter seems to have shouldered the most impact. Logistics services are the main reason for the delays experienced in the supply chain. Hence, countries like Saudi Arabia are on the lookout for ways to foster localization.

These countries want to encourage local production and continue sourcing products from various countries to mitigate any disruptions. China and India are the dominators in global production; therefore, it will be challenging for some countries to reorient their supply chains immediately to meet global demand, but it will be vital for long term goals.

For example, Mexico relies on India and China for between 90 to 95 percent of its Active Pharmaceutical Ingredients (APIs). Such dependency, combined with the present lack of international air connections, makes it even more impossible to enable immediate restructuring.

Countries with direct flights to India and China could be able to maintain their supply chains relatively. The lack of direct air ties with the world's significant producers is bound to make Mexicans and Latin Americans suffer from the scarcity of many critical pharmaceutical products. Albeit, due to the restricted transport options, there may be delays in some regions of the supply chain, several border authorities have taken steps to ensure that drugs reach the end-user as soon as possible.

For example, Dubai's customs have launched new practices to allow the rapid clearing of medical supplies and pharmaceutical products. The Customs Service is looking forward to managing higher volumes of critical supplies through advanced technology and specialist gears at its control centers. All these networks, chains, hiccups, emergencies, supplies, shortages, delays, and possible solutions fall in line with ideas in recreating modern healthcare systems with a more enhanced logistic module. Before the advent of coronavirus, medical distribution chains were far from perfect.

Now the healthcare crises have just revealed how much work needs to be done to handle such catastrophes in the future successfully. There is evidence that points to the possibility of COVID 19, leading to more long-lasting effects. Many supply chain experts believe that China could risk losing its central position on many global supply networks in Brazil, Mexico, and other emerging markets in Southeast Asia.

There is a two-fold reason for this: the initial shock from China-centric supply chains, brought on by widespread industrial hibernation across the country. The second reason is that the trade war between the United States and China has already left companies with no choice but to look elsewhere.

COVID 19 has accelerated American companies' trend to realign their supply chains with countries closer to home. They are also diversifying them to reduce future exposure to risks by relocating to Asian nations such as Malaysia, Vietnam, Thailand, and Indonesia. Companies most likely to consider relocating their operations are electronic, textiles, and renewable energy sectors.

According to Citibank analysis, investors would consider looking to the Southeast Asia trade block to make things significantly less overbearing in such crises. Additionally, some businesses hailing from Taiwan are anticipated to relocate some parts of their supply chains to ASEAN (Association of Southeast Asian Nations) with the new Southbound Policy. A possible sign of this is a broader trend of nations relocating their facilities in the Asia-Pacific.

Before the pandemic, foreign banks' lending to China was falling, while ASEAN recorded a 6.9 percent year-on-year credit expansion. According to February 2020 report from equities and derivatives, brokerage companies from the broader economic pack of Asia had already begun adopting a China strategy. Such firms include Japan's Honda and Toyota as well as South Korea's Samsung.

The strategy is an indication that they intend to diversify their supply chains regionally. These companies are trying to offset future risks from operating only within China. Covid-19 is also affecting clinical trials.

In general, approximately 20 percent of studies are conducted in China, where the virus originated. According to the United States clinical trials database, nearly 500 trials are conducted at sites in Wuhan. Beyond site issues, there are other forms of delays in current and planned trails, which are likely to occur even as the epidemic makes its way across the planet. Halts that reduce patient enrollment, patients dropping out of trials, or the non-compliances with study procedures are anticipated.

The Food and Drug Administration (FDA) should engage firms to solve the problems in bolstering new medical supplies. The long and short-term impacts of coronavirus on supply chains, clinical trials, and the general sector of pharma and medical device companies show less stability of full materialization. When the SAR epidemic of 2013 sang its terrifying song, the demand for medical supplies went up within a short period. During the period of the outbreak, there was low sustainability.

If one considers the hidden and robust transmission of the novel coronavirus, undoubtedly, the outbreak's duration might be longer than envisaged. The disturbing deficit in frontline medical services calls for the hospitalization of only diagnosed patients in severe conditions, repeating what happened during the previous pandemics. The only evidence that can be garnered right now is symptomatic and supportive treatment. Devices that support the respiratory system, like atomizers, oxygen generators, and ventilators, among other life-support machines, comprises current essential clinical treatment for now.

Due to this reality, the need for diagnosis instruments and life-aiding devices remains overwhelming than everything else. To restore a balance between supply and demand, most governments launched an emergency approval process to register and distribute medical devices urgently needed to prevent and contain the virus.

It can be difficult to make rapid changes in a supply chain or manufacturing changes due to the medical device industry's highly regulated nature. It may not be manageable in the short term. However, given the uncertain duration of the impact, it may be time to take a good look at anticipating potential transitions as we see longer-term effects on the supply chain.

There might be an opportunity to partner with other regulatory agencies when critical devices are needed, as explained above. Specific quality system regulation (QSR) requirements could be waived to mitigate shortages and ensure availability. Thus, Companies should be allowed to manufacture devices that would be eligible for emergency use, provided safety of the end-user is granted. Based on conventional wisdom, the steady demand for medical products and procedures will insulate MedTech companies from the current economic disruption to display stability in these uncertain times. As the medical device industry goes through unchartered territory, supply chain managers should develop more effective ways to demonstrate their expertise.

Delivery schedules from Original Equipment Manufacturers (OEMs) might change because they are also dealing with market disruptions. The best option is for suppliers not to complain about or ignore the uncertainty; they must devise plans to prove to consumers that societal disruptions will not affect their manufacturing volume.

CHAPTER FIVE

Rights of Fulfilment During Pandemics

Due to the COVID-19 pandemic, it might be impossible for organizations to meet their contractual obligations. Below are real-life scenarios about the pandemic and its consequence on the rights of fulfillment.

Scenario #1: As a supplier with a contractual obligation to supply goods to customers. However, logistics issues (caused by border restrictions) have delayed the supply of raw material from a subcontractor. Thus, I cannot supply goods to customers on time. Despite the pandemic, do I still have the legal obligation to fulfill my contractual undertakings? We can consider an epidemic to be a force majeure.

Based on the situation described, different situations may arise when a debtor cannot fulfill his contractual obligation in time. An essential part of the contract (by contractual provision or by the transaction) is the fulfillment deadline. If it is not fulfilled, then the agreement is terminated when the deadline expires. However, the creditor may retain the contract should the creditor inform the debtor (upon expiration and without delay) that the contract's performance is a requirement - note that this is not obligatory.

If this obligation is not satisfied, the creditor is obliged to cancel the contract. Bear in mind that if the requirement is fulfilled within a reasonable new deadline, the creditor may re-consider. The creditor may also still request an extension even if the deadline for fulfillment of obligation is not an essential part of the contract. It is within the debtor's right to fulfill the requirement regardless of the expiration deadline. However, the debtor must be given a sufficient subsequent period for fulfillment should the creditor terminate the contract after the deadline. These deadlines are taken as legal standards because there is no definition for a reasonable or appropriate timeframe. Thus, they are interpreted based on specific circumstances regarding each situation.

When the creditor suffers liability for damage due to delayed or default fulfillment of contractual obligations, the debtor will not be answerable to such liability for damage provided he can prove that circumstances he could not avoid, eliminate or prevent after entering the contract is his reason for defaulting or delaying the fulfillment of his obligations. Thus, the current COVID-19 pandemic can be considered a force majeure. However, this must be proven on a case-by-case basis. That is, the presence of a pandemic does not make the debtor's failure to fulfill his obligation a foregone conclusion.

Scenario #2: *I entered into an agreement before COVID-19, but there has been significant deterioration to my position, and I cannot deliver the contract supplies timely because the deal has become highly disadvantageous for me. Can I renegotiate the terms of the agreement, or how should I address the situation?*

This situation may require the application of the rebus Sic Stantibus (the change of circumstance clause). According to this law, if certain circumstances arise after the contract's conclusion, then the part that cannot fulfill obligations or cannot accomplish the contract's purpose may seek the contract's cancellation.

Such certain circumstances are:

- The difficulty for either of the parties to fulfill the terms of the obligation
- It is impossible to achieve the purpose of the contract because of these difficulties

These circumstances are proof that:

- The expectations of the contracting parties about the contract cannot be met
- It would be unfair to maintain this contract in its current form.

However, if the following situations are obtainable, a contractual party does not have the right to request contract termination.

Situation #1: It was necessary to consider these circumstances at the time of the contract's conclusion. While an epidemic is not recognized under this obligation, there may be exceptions. For example, did the party conclude the contract before the declaration of the outbreak in his region or after its confirmation?

Situation #2: The circumstance's existence after the deadline's expiration for fulfilling the obligation. It is important to note that the agreement to modify certain parts of the contract makes it possible for the other party to leave the contract valid.

Once the above conditions are met, the new situation is an opportunity to raise contract modification. When there is no consent between the parties, the court considers specific statutory circumstances before deciding to terminate or amend the contract.

Scenario #3: This pandemic only makes it possible for me to fulfill my obligations partially. For example, I can only supply 50% of the items in the contract. Is the contract still in existence? What are the provisions of the contract performance when delivery is challenging but not entirely impossible?

The critical question in this scenario is the volume of obligations that can be satisfied. For instance, failure to satisfy a small part of the requirement cannot lead to the contract's termination. However, if a pandemic or a similar event makes it impossible to fulfill a significant portion of the obligation and the partial fulfillment does not meet the other party's needs, he may terminate the contract. If not, the agreement is still valid, and there is a significant reduction in the creditor's obligation. When it becomes extremely difficult (but not impossible) to fulfill contractual obligations, it might be necessary to consider applying the rebus Sic Santibus clause.

Scenario #4: Are there different rules when the contract is with a foreign entity?

The states' law regulates the rules described above. Thus, as mentioned earlier, the provisions apply to a specific contractual relationship provided it conforms with specific contracts and standards of private international law. It is also possible to use the united nations convention on contracts for the international sale of goods (CISG) under specific circumstances as 89 countries signed it.

These rules specify details of the relationship concerning the purchase of goods - for example, force majeure conditions for discharge from liability, the right to report such conditions, and the effects of contract cancellation.

Global Challenges in Fulfillment Agreements

As the COVID-19 situation expands globally, its effects on the Chinese and Italian consumer products industries make it possible to predict certain factors that impact consumer products companies in other countries. A company's product category is arguably the most significant factor. It is no longer a secret that consumers in areas affected by the virus have been hoarding essential pantry and household items (exceptionally packaged shelf-stable food and disease-prevention products).

The spread of the disease has led to the emergence of four main category archetypes:

1. Panic-buy for disaster-preparedness categories. These categories include medical supplies, instant meals, hand sanitizer, masks, and disinfectants. The massive demand for these categories has far outweighed its supply. Hence, there is a speedy turnover and constant out-of-stocks.
2. High volume stocking of daily essentials goods in the pantry. These essentials include bottled water, regular hygiene products, shelf-stable groceries, infant food, and formula. There are below-average stock levels with face constrained supply.
3. Limited short supply of discretionary household products such as pet care, personal care, snack foods, soft drinks, and traditional dairy.
4. Severe reduction in non-essentials and luxury products. The products here include alcoholic beverages, confectionery, luxury beauty, skincare, and cosmetics. There has been a

rapid collapse in demand for these categories. Alcoholic beverages are more subjected to reliance on-trade sales (until temporary closures and social-distancing measures are suspended).

The increased at-home consumption and the stock-up effect has affected traditional grocery retail channels greatly. Consumers' desire to stock up has massively accelerated consumer adoption of online channels. Consequently, it has minimized close human contact and public exposure. The logistic difficulties created by the rapid and unforeseen increase in demand for online food items, an emerging medium in most markets, will, unfortunately, be met in most businesses.

For example, in the United States, fulfillment players, such as the traditional 1 to 2-hour delivery window of Amazon Prime now, have been expanding in some areas to almost 24 hours, and the availability of InstaCart is already limited. As customers have a mandatory quarantine in some regions, while others do not go into the public to prevent infections, out-of-home outlets have declined rapidly.

This pronounced decrease in on-site sales had two effects:

1. Market products businesses that are primarily dependent on home networks have been adversely affected.

2. Distributors and wholesalers on these networks have dire consequences.

Most face liquidity constraints already and may soon announce bankruptcy or closure. The spikes and dips in demand for products of the consumer product companies have led to intense stress. Thus, it requires these companies to quickly adapt their production strategies, transportation and distribution, critical account management, and marketing.

In the wake of COVID-19, the most significant challenge for consumer products companies is supply chain considerations. Supply continuity poses a severe problem due to ongoing health concerns, quarantined workers, and forced extended holidays, especially for companies whose primary raw materials suppliers reside in profoundly affected areas. Also, packaging companies and other smaller suppliers immediately faced cash flow issues, which add more pressure to their lean operations.

In some categories, their supply chains were pushed beyond capacity by a combination of panic-buying and production constraints. The short-term essence of their contingency plans has stepped up their challenges for most consumer goods companies.

Few businesses will expand their contingency plans for the first quarter of 2020 to incidents such as the COVID-19 pandemic.

Most of the lean manufacturing and supply chain strategies also demand that inventories be available at any time for three months. The situation is worsened by increasing inbound and outbound supply chain challenges and logistical bottlenecks, which restricted travel networks. With these constraints, some suppliers could not meet the soaring demands for staple items.

As the shelves become empty, panic-buying will increase, leading to a vicious cycle of corruption. The early days of lockdown in Italy resulted in an inbound supply risk because carriers willing to transport into the "red zones" (profoundly affected areas) have been grossly insufficient. Hence, warehouses in such areas faced outbound supply risk. Apart from consumer products companies, most third-party distributors and wholesalers face similar turnover and inventory challenges. Low-demand categories proved vulnerable to oversupply, while huge-demand product categories were sensitive to insufficient supply, leading to cash flow problems.

Another consequence of the COVID-19 outbreak has been a tenser relationship between consumer products companies and retailers, usually in disagreement over trade negotiations, demand planning, and supply issues.

Most in-person talks have become transactional since these negotiations now take place via voice calls or video calls. A growing concern is less-rigorous demand planning since out-of-stocks and overstocks are now unacceptable to retailers. The focus of crucial account manager/retailer buyer conversations is now on fundamental, survival-mode supply concerns instead of standard pricing, promotion, and trade spending discussions.

Companies have also had to adapt to consumer traffic changes by shifting most of their marketing activities offline to online. Most consumer products companies have suspended or called off their planned marketing campaigns, particularly in-store and out-of-home events or activations.

The outbreak is also changing consumers' attention and media consumption marketing channels and content. Daytime media audiences are growing as more people remain at home. The desire to stay connected and up-to-date on COVID-19 coverage has increased. Many brands are now adjusting their strategies to suit these changes. This shift in strategy involves more spending on digital ads, news, and health-education platforms. During these turbulent times, brands are also adjusting their messaging to increase awareness and sensitivity.

Consumers cannot afford to sit and wait for everything to flip to normal since this global pandemic is unpredictable. They must respond fast to this new shock to business. Depending on the virus' rate in markets, planning and response should be in three pivotal phases:

Phase 1: The virus is already known, but not many people have been affected. Despite normal daily activities, most consumers are now stocking up on essentials and reducing discretionary spending. This phase is already underway in most countries. Consumer products companies playing non-essential categories must be ready to adjust to weaker demand. At the same time, those in essential groups must develop a plan to address a likely surge in demand. This time must be spent on production. The companies must apply urgent plans that can prevent escalation into the next phase.

Phase 2: The prevalence of the virus in markets and authorities have taken strict measures such as lockdowns, closure of schools, public places, and implementation of quarantines. Thus, there are labor shortages, considerable disruptions to supply, demand, operations, and logistical flows. For many Asian and European markets, phase two is their current reality.

Phase 3: Recovery and beyond - gradually return to normality. This phase involves significant alteration to competitive positions and relationships with retail customers and changes to consumers' share of wallet and buying options. The checklist below can help leadership teams to develop a short-term multipurpose response:

Checklist #1: An Emergency Response Team

- Set up a cross-functional emergency response that will work closely with the chief executive, the chief financial officer, and the principal task officer. This is like having a virtual war room office given the team's global nature, office closures, and social distancing. This team may agree on some principles and processes as the situation intensifies, and urgent decision-making is required. Then, for speed and effectiveness, they can move to more localized decision making. Apart from having direct access to key executives, empower the team to make recommendations that cover the rapid assessment of risks in vital areas of the workforce, supply inventory, and consumer sentiment.

- Indicate exact daily duties for the team in these three key areas:
  a. Reporting internal essential performance and indicators
  b. Tracking, reviewing, and adjusting the emergency response.
  c. Managing internal and external communications.
- Set up relevant local emergency response teams. This setup can be based on a distribution center or function, manufacturing facility, business unit, country, or region.

- A team member should be solely responsible for scanning relevant information about the virus's spread and its effects on actions by other consumer products companies, consumer demand, and retailer reactions.

Checklist #2: Protection is Utmost Priority

Protecting the health and safety of its employees, customers, supplies, and other partners should be the core obligation of any consumer products company. The emergency response team must recommend and communicate necessary actions and involve everyone in the coordinated plan.

Ideally, companies must do the following task:

- Ensure compliance with the latest guidance by communicating with local authorities and speedily providing their recommendations throughout the organization's department.
- Emphasize the importance of workers staying at home when they feel ill and screening or sending individuals to their homes when necessary.
- Enforce frequent hand washing and surface sanitization rules.
- Equip employees with appropriate personal protection equipment (such as gloves, masks, and disinfecting wipes) to effectively do their job. This is more relevant to manufacturing personnel (to prevent product contamination) and

sales teams (to prevent exposure from customer or store visits).

- If the infection is rapidly spreading in a location, co-located teams must work from two or more office locations.

- For business-critical executives or functional leaders, identify and nominate backup options quickly. Hence, another person can step up to replace an infected person.

- Certain business-critical functions might necessitate a "red and blue team" approach. Core functions are split into two teams who alternate the days. They go into the office and can work from home or within the office in separate units. If a blue team member gets sick, the red team can still function until the other team return from their isolation or quarantine.

- Cancel gatherings of not more than 20 people whose operations are not critical.

- Consider for secondary work arrangements for high-risk employees.

- Prepare for work-from-home requirements and put in place technology solutions so that employees can work regardless of their location.

- Stop non-essential travel. Employees should replace in-person customer visits with video or conference calls (for example, crucial account managers), and salesforces should do likewise to prevent unnecessary store visits.

- Implement formal advice on how to clean frequently deep used facility areas such as HVAC ducts, air conditioners, air purifiers, elevators, meeting rooms, and bathrooms.
- Short-term closure of cafeterias and canteens - stop the provision of shared food and refreshments.
- Eliminate third-party office visits.

Checklist #3: Review to Alter Production Plan and Inventory Management

- Secure continuity of supply by developing contingency plans. Apart from making sure that factory and warehouse personnel are available for daily work, take precautionary measures and enact safety protocols to protect employee health.
- Determine and address the supply chain's weakest links (in order of priority) in terms of resiliency - access to transportation, health/sanitary supplies, warehouse space, packaging, raw materials, and workforce.
- **Immediate production plans based on certain adjustments:**
  a. Product category exposure: Increase high-demand categories proportionally and reduce production for groups that might likely experience a short-term decline. Limit production range to the popular "hero" SKUs and pack

sizes. Thus, there would be no interruption to production lines, and it is easier to sustain demand.

b. Channel mix (distribution) exposure: For channels with an increase in demand (warehouse clubs, supermarkets, hypermarkets, and online markets), hasten the production of SKUs and formats. Reduce production for products with intense exposure to out-of-home channels. Shift mixing of products and packages ideal for at-home consumption.

c. Analyze ways to use diversification of manufacturing for risk arbitrage measures: prevent interruption from business-related tasks by splitting production across countries, plants, and teams in cases of rapid outbreak/transmission. Also, put in place business continuity measures and utilize flexible production measures. Thus, total production will not stop whether there is prolonged quarantine. Implementation of such plans might involve the forward deployment of inventory and temporary production facilities or warehouses.

d. Where necessary, use co-manufacturing and broader manufacturing ecosystem as spare capacity. Intimate third-party manufacturers of enhanced sanitary precautions and make sure that they do likewise.

e. Be closer to raw material suppliers and carefully observe any increasing lead times. Develop contingency plans that suitably replace raw materials/input sourcing if raw material production facilities stop working altogether. Assess and adapt production and supply for all tiers of suppliers, including suppliers' suppliers. Do not make the same mistake that most of the leadership teams do. Be prepared for the complications that may arise from lower-order suppliers.

f. Increase stock levels for items with enormous demands and move inventory to the market very quickly.

g. Closely monitor stock levels and fulfillment. Shut down automatic replenishment and other algorithms that do not fit current demand patterns.

Checklist #4: Improve logistics flexibility

- Get realistic details of potential lockdown areas from the authorities and develop plans to deliver to such areas.

- Re-evaluate transport and delivery plan that suit quick stock delivery to stores. Tactics will need to be checked. For example, compare delivery via distribution centers with direct store delivery to determine the option that will give the best results.

- Stop planned deliveries of non-essential categories to free up freight capacity. Then, enforce minimum order quantities for freight aggressively. When short on capacity, work with retailers to determine the availability of near-term backhaul or customer pickup opportunities.

- Leverage collective capacity with logistics providers and even competitors. Explore other distribution options such as third-party on-demand logistics providers or less-then-truckload (LTL) flexible distributors.

- For different warehouses and distribution centers, use separate logistics providers. This segmentation of transport flows will mitigate transmission risks.

- Ensure strict adherence of delivery fleets and other external logistics partners to hygiene standards, including trucks and vans' sanitization.

- Be swift with making logistics decisions. For example, move inventory out of customer warehouses to places where it is urgently needed or move them around the network.

Checklist #5: Adjust to demand but remain close to customers

- Customers will be expecting new levels of proximity and more frequent communication. Hence, account managers must be available for real-time, spontaneous customer conversations.

- The focus of key account management should now be continuity of supply rather than traditional buying negotiations. This might involve temporary compromises for the most critical categories and customers. For example, relaxing accounts receivable terms. It might include short-term adjustments for retailers such as in-full fines and lifting on-time.

- Resolve pain points and bottlenecks quickly by working within agile multifunctional teams (which might be virtual meetups where in-person meetups are no longer possible). Then, provide creative, resourceful solutions to clients. For instance, adjustment of production plans to transmit customer order information to SOP quickly. Discuss alternative delivery mechanisms with the logistics team to distribute inventory to customers in the affected areas. Increase product availability by reaching an agreement with the manufacturing team for them to produce larger batches of specific SKUs.

- Make online retail quicker. The categories that are moving positively toward online during this pandemic will remain there for the foreseeable future. It might be necessary to start using fit-for-purpose pack sizes for online sales. Some brands might use this period as an opportunity to embrace online channels fully. A few will even begin to use auto-re-plenishment features.

- When using online retail, be watchful of third-party sellers who might want to take advantage of the situation and start reselling items at highly exorbitant prices. The curbing of such price extortion swiftly leveraging strong customer relationships.

- Focus on more significant pack types for relevant categories. Alternatively, adjust to suit purchase patterns through bulk purchase.

- Determine pricing and promotions. Prevent unnecessary burning of budges by resetting promotion levels at a specific category more than averages. Consider stopping promotional activities for sensitive product categories like hand sanitizer, medical supplies, and disinfectant (the government in some countries might set the prices for these items).

- Instead of spending time and energy on pricing/promotion conversations, use this time and energy to discuss broader supply-focused topics. Tending to the success of often-vulnerable retailers and sustaining stock during the crisis can be profitable for future customer relationships.

- Ease the pains of wholesalers and on-trade customers by staying close to them. Consumer goods companies who serve the on-trade channel are in an awkward position. They must balance conservative credit policies to extend a lifeline to the out-of-home customers and distributors. These policies are meant to minimize future losses while the out-of-home customers and distributors might soon be facing bad debt fallouts. Use this period to analyze customer networks to determine relationships thoroughly. The cut off will be the worst come possible. Also, consider mom-and-pop shops that might be at risk from cash flow shortages.

"Focus on the customers who absolutely love your product, focus on the features required to attract and retain those customers, and focus on the team that's mission-critical to delivering your service in turbulent times."

- Andrew Hoag, CEO of Teampay

Checklist #6: Adjust marketing strategies and messaging

- Ensure that new touch points indicate the new shifts within the customer landscape. Replace out-of-home and physical media with online and digital media. Reduce in-person and on-trade activations and events. Shift to less traditional but more relevant avenues that reflect changing consumer behavior, such as health channels, education networks, and gaming.

- There should be less focus on non-mission-critical marketing spending and activities. Thus, there will be a budget for mission-critical operations and short-term improvements, which results in cash and working capital.

- Content and messaging must be timely, relevant, and appropriate to suit the pandemic narrative. Even if one does not play within the space, broader health and safety messages are a sign of commitment to consumers. Stop campaigns that are not relevant during the crisis as it can harm brand equity.

- Make quick mental decisions about online marketing spending. Avoid advertising that can result in low (or no) ROI by emphasizing close collaboration among marketing, supply chain, and essential account management functions. For instance, stop promoting Amazon products that are already sold-out on the site. Clorox is an example of such a product. They are reducing advertising per product supply.

Checklist #7: Observe cash flow and capital during times of crisis

Thus, eliminate or hold on to non-essential or non-strategic projects. Consumer products companies must take this seriously since a squeeze effect is possible. For example, as players in the spiking categories build workforce redundancy, they will experience a short-term impact on costs.

Still, it will increase logistical flows, accelerate production, and ensure continued operations. Customers may not even pay them immediately after the release of funds. Players with exposure to declining channels or decelerating categories will experience a rapid reduction in demand and difficulties in receiving payment from customers facing a cash crunch. It is possible to have various working capital enhancements, such as measures that can improve cash conversion.

For example, increasing inventory turns by reducing the prices of slow movers. Where necessary, companies can cancel training on non-critical operations to reduce their overhead costs.

There will likely be disruptions of better deals, which might alter opportunities in some cases.

Establish contingency plans and varying valuations by coordinating with the investment bankers/deal team to advance closure dates. Watch for reasonable goals that would dramatically affect the markets following the outbreak within the same period. Stay close to stakeholders to determine circumstances that can lead to large cost-reduction, especially in the broader economic climate.

Checklist #8: Communication and collaboration is key

Supporting society through a crisis such as the COVID-19 outbreak is a vital role of consumer products companies. Hence, senior marketing executives must keep open lines of communication with relevant authorities in their markets. This might involve being conversant with the latest government laws about curtailing panic-buying and shortages or possible lockdown areas subject to logistical constraints.

When products are available regardless of the odds, it creates a sense of goodwill. However, if companies do not follow the recommended precautions and health guidelines, their reputation may suffer severely.

There must be communication to assure workers' safety, emphasizing the necessary measures to protect personnel. Regardless of their rank, all employees prefer to hear important internal news from the management rather than hearing it as rumors. Employees want the feeling of company empathy regarding the personal cost of the pandemic.

Checklist #9: Take it beyond business

During this unprecedented situation, brands play a vital humanitarian role and might need to look beyond their business to demonstrate empathy to those in distress. Short-term marketing messages that underline their commitment to helping during this crisis are necessary, but they are insufficient. Thus, brands must act and respond through more violent means.

Donations to hospitals and medical institutions are simple and popular. Several brands in China have taken this step. For instance, LVMH (a multinational luxury group) has already donated $2.3 million to the Chinese red cross foundation to combat medical supplies shortage. Estee Lauder, L'Oreal, and Kering are brands that have made similar donations. In Italy, Grocer Esselunga donated 2.5 million euros to Italian hospitals and has provided free online delivery to customers above 65 years of age (the population who are the most susceptible to this virus).

An additional step is for companies to provide tangible disaster support and relief by leveraging their resources and capabilities. As part of its disaster relief efforts, Anheuser-Busch has provided emergency drinking water in the last 30 years. They have provided more than 80 million water cans in the United States alone. Hence, one positive contribution can result in deep loyalty and brand equity in the long-term.

Pointing Paths to Recovery

It can be a struggle to keep abreast of the immediate challenges during this moment of strain. It is even harder to focus on the medium or long-term. Nevertheless, during this COVID-19 crisis, leadership teams in consumer products must recognize the need not to lose sight of the broader goals. They must plan for phase 3 - the eventual recovery. At the same time, it may take some time before normality returns. Phase 3 is necessary to prepare and welcome back the staff and return to the pre-crisis situation gradually.

Companies' utmost priority should still be the creation of a healthy workplace environment. Disclose steps take to sustain safety and hygiene. Then, add the additional measures as you work with suppliers and distributors. Use this pandemic experience to fortify business against future epidemics, pandemics, terrorist attacks, economic downturns, or natural disasters.

Conduct a post-mortem of the problem so that lessons can be learned. Write down resources and teams dedicated to managing the crisis gradually. Systemize approach for a similar crisis to activate an emergency response team promptly. Recovery also entails resetting and restarting the 2020 plan with new operational plans, forecasts of budgets, and objectives. Apart from that, part of companies 3-year plan must now include critical actions:

- Use customer and market data review to analyze aspects where the company profited or lost market share during COVID-19. The report should include ways the company's highest-value customers survived the crisis. Then, nurture those relationships by identifying necessary actions.

- Adjust to post-crisis demand by rebalancing stock levels.

- Reactivate demand by creating commercial revitalization plans.

- Update the target partnership list and identify opportunities in the value chain.

- Enforce regular cost improvement strategies, particularly in categories whose anticipated recovery seems slow.

- In the long-term, companies should use this period to propel them to build long-term capabilities. Thus, they can prepare for a future crisis and serve the customer and consumer needs with greater efficiency and effectiveness.

- Make all efforts to ensure a resilient supply chain. This involves the identification of additional supply sources and utilizing technology that makes flexible capacity planning possible. Invest in improving automation, production nodes, and distributed inventory.

- Monitor the end-to-end supply chain using a central tower. This tower should be a decision-making platform for a real-time, integrated, and omniscient supply chain. Thus, making predictive/prescriptive analytics and end-to-end visibility possible. It increases efficiency without having to implement any short-term widespread structural changes. Over time, it allows for critical visibility into structural adjustment options and creates a step-change impact.

- Improve knowledge of "new retail." Now brands can become omnichannel leaders by activating and flexing commercial muscles. This involves monitoring consumers' migration to new touch points and fully delivering on the "anywhere, anytime" premise. Explore all aspects of digital marketing, such as route-to-market, marketing, and product levers.

- Analyze the complete route-to-market models. Instead of a more agile ecosystem, experiment with fewer layers of distributors. Then, prioritize must-win relationships and closely identify possible gaps to fill by re-examining customer and distributor network.
- Focus on building digital capabilities. Such as e-commerce, marketing, and new working methods.

Inventory must be moved to hospitals to keep inventory fresh and made for the emergency inventory. Each new order will build a new batch of equipment and shipping continuously. Make sure not enough equipment is available. The concept is that a group of qualified personnel will be formed in hospitals for a few weeks each year to retain their ability to maintain their expertise and to train on new equipment to supplement regular staff during a significant crisis.

In this sense, we need to have trained personnel who will require a medical "National Guard." These strategies can seem drastic, but global crises, such as Covid-19, may warn that traditional approaches are not appropriate. In times of crisis, we are preparing for oil and arms shortages. It is now painfully clear that medical supplies like other life-supporting products are just as essential.

CHAPTER SIX

Re-engineering During Pandemics

During a pandemic, engineers are attempting to redesign equipment to combat a massive increase in demand and stalled supply chains to produce the needed medical gears without using specialized factories. Researchers at academic institutions have established clubs for D.I.Y(do-it-yourself) enthusiasts. The do-it-yourself approach is most apparent in the creation of face masks. Enthusiasts are teaching amateurs how to sew their washable coverings by providing them with various designs and instructions. While some have donated these masks to hospitals, such unofficial gear can only be a last resort in a medical setting.

Research has proven that these homemade facial protections are less effective than professionally produced surgical masks, but they can reduce microbes' spread. The difference in effectiveness is because homespun masks are made from untested fabrics, while surgical masks are made from materials that can halt the virus-dropping droplets more effectively. Some manufacturing companies have begun to make more impermeable clothing and masks. The process and results of manufacturing gears such as face shields are too time-consuming and are not suitable for mass production. Engineers have developed an alternative approach of making facial shields produced en masse by 3-D printers and laser cutters.

Facial Protection

Any commercial die cutter, laser cutter, or water jet can use an origami-style design (an open-source design from the MASK project). A summary of this design involves hand-folding a flat sheet of plastic into an appropriate 3-dimensional shape. Researchers from organizations such as the Massachusetts Institute of technology and Duke University health system have developed and tested their face-shield prototypes. While M.I.T and MASK project's shield have similar designs., Duke health's design is made from a 3-D printed headband. The most crucial point is that all these new shields can be produced from conventional machines. Most manufacturers' spaces, labs, and production facilities that do not usually make medical equipment have laser cutters, die cutters, and 3-D printers.

Most of these mini-engineering teams require partners to manufacture these devices. Such partners can be a small shop that cuts out pieces of paper into shapes or large factories with roller die cutters, producing hundreds of thousands of shields per day. The manufactured devices from these distributed manufacturing models are sent to a central hub for quality control and sanitization before being distributed to hospitals. Despite never having done this scale of distributed manufacturing, the business community amazingly and rapidly sorted out the supply chains.

Filter-agnostic Face Shield

Though distributed manufacturing requires re-engineering equipment, it has the advantage of speed. With this re-engineered equipment, items can be produced without specialized devices such as 3-D printers. Even with that, some of these new designs do not meet strict medical standards. Regardless of their scarcity, medical standards cannot be lowered for specific items such as N95 respirators.

While a few viral particles can squeeze through surgical masks, the material can still halt droplets. This is especially important since viral particles can fill the air when doctors ventilate critically-ill coronavirus patients. Thus, medical professionals put on N95 respirators to protect themselves in such situations. Apart from fitting closely to the skin, these masks block 95% of tiny particles and only admit air through a dense filter. Nevertheless, it still allows individuals to breathe effortlessly. Spun polypropylene is the primary material for the filter in an N95;the problem is that the material scarce.

An alternative to the N95 is a filter-agnostic face shield. It has been designed, prototyped, and tested. The 3-D printed base of the MASK project respirator makes it tightly fitted to the face. The respirator consists of a front-grate having filtering materials like the particle specification of the N95, which allows the passage of air. Tests are still ongoing on this product for filtering and breathability. Since the food and drug administration now allows U.S. organizations to use alternatives (such as KN95s) to N95s, the MASK project's device can also serve as a substitute for shortages of comparable devices.

Ventilator Re-design

Ventilators, just like N95 respirators, must conform to high medical manufacturing standards. Ventilators provide oxygen for COVID-19 patients when the amount of oxygen in their blood drops to dangerous levels. However, despite manufacturers increasing their production rate, these sophisticated, expensive devices are still in short supply worldwide.

Drawing inspiration from the squeeze bag, researchers are still exploring the use of a single-use ventilator. Health workers manually use squeeze bags to control a patient's breathing in emergencies. They combine such a device with an oxygen supply and an apparatus that automates the squeeze and release process.

By doing so, the infected person can breathe for a more extended period, just like when using a ventilator. In the UK, this ventilator substitute is in its second phase of testing before approval from the drugs and healthcare products regulatory agency (this agency is the UK's equivalent to the F.D.A. in the United States).

The open-source design for this medical device would be by Smith Nephew manufacturers once the developers receive the go-ahead. While there are other emergency ventilator prototypes, most of them are discarded after single-patient use. Also, it lacks alarms and monitoring equipment compared to full-scale ventilators. Using this type of equipment from the MASK project, companies can scale up emergency ventilator designs more quickly.

Doorknobs

To mitigate the issues related to areas where employees re-peatedly use the surfaces, the Gemba walk concept could prevent employees from COVID-19   infections. For example, elbows hooks could replace doorknobs; the refrigerator handles could be re-placed with foot pull and change in the toilet designs to enable a push or flushing using the forearm.

The Role of Clinical Engineering

The danger of a lack of sufficient facilities for patients receiving COVID-19 treatment is distressing. These facilities can sometimes be adjusted, altered, reconfigured, or even slightly changed to be used in different setups. Several general or special test sites are designed to support patients with this virus for diagnosis. In addition to research, various healthcare organizations build or use segregated areas where patients are released to clean beds and combat the flooding in their hospitals while helping the most in need. Such isolated areas may not have the necessary technology to meet the clinical equipment requirements to treat COVID-19 patients. Consequently, a confident strategic improvisation between leadership, IT, and clinical engineering is required.

All organizations, including oversight from third parties, arrangements through original instruments manufacturers, and internal healthcare development programs, have interests and abilities to endorse medicinal and surgical instruments based on different factors.

The hope is such organizations will have the knowledge, skills, resources, energy, and ability to support and help in the COVID-19 crisis, irrespective of who manages such technologies. To strategize rapidly and aid throughout the strategic goals during this period, the company must communicate clearly. Healthcare engineering will play a vital role in supporting the organization by supplying assistance if appropriate and in every way possible. Such services should involve helping to convert single rooms into double rooms at the discretion of the leadership. Help to move, and set up medical monitors, beds, applications, and contact nurses, thermometers, fans.

Clinical engineering has now been influential in training healthcare workers and designing clinical strategies. Specific organizations are assessing or managing COVID-19 cases in hospitals or hospital clinics. Clinical engineering can help to configure medical instruments to incorporate data collection into electronic health records in such environments. Hardware mounting, data capture configuration, network link activation, and wireless networking is required. In certain instances, the data is collected, preserved, and only submitted later.

These places are not currently equipped; therefore, the specifications of facilities or equipment installed in these areas need clinical evaluation. Hospital improvements should also work with clinical stakeholders to address questions before programs are moved. Some have said that using a stationary imaging system is not advised for other patients and staff because of cleaning processes and possible virus exposure. The usage of portable devices for those who use these services is recommended.

Digital Health Tech on Clinical Trials

While most governments rely on social distancing measures to prevent COVID-19 infections, it is now time for health organizations to step up the use of telemedicine tools. The world health organization recommends the optimization of delivery options. Introducing telemedicine into clinical services enhances decision support tools and reduces face-to-face interactions through self-isolation and online healthcare workers as a solution to the board.

The severity of the pandemic is contagion to the extent to which clinical trials have generally been halted in many scientific areas. Conducting clinical trials even for COVID 19 has become a dilemma for the following reasons:

- Participants and Healthcare personnel remain in isolation, while some are affected by the process.
- Overwhelmed Healthcare facilities and limited resources to coordinate participants from different locations and systemic discrepancies have led to testing applications' reprioritization.

One of the alternatives now discussed by most expects is expanding on digital health technology. Experts believe this will lead to the transformation of clinical trials procedure that will inadvertently involve virtual trials. The FDA has updated intuitive guidance that balances maintaining regulatory compliance, safety conditions for trial participants and reducing the risk during the trials. The guidelines acknowledge a few deviations in the standard protocol regarding remote visits and options that might involve telemedicine.

It is challenging for sponsors and clinical expects because such studies' feasible nature has never involved remote monitoring. Despite support from the Federal Communication Commission (FCC) and other investments to aid remote monitoring of patients in hospitals and healthcare systems, there are still doubts about how the space for clinical trials could be managed.

Many experts acknowledge the need to pivot to digital and remote site monitoring because of the enormous benefits, ranging from cost reduction, efficiency, and more accessibility to collected data.

"Aptar Pharma has a well-established position worldwide in drug delivery technologies across the whole value chain, collaborating with Aptar will help us expand and speed up clinical application and commercialization of Sonmol's innovative products. I look forward to more in-depth and innovative exploration and collaboration between Aptar and Sonmol in the field of drug and disease digital management in China and worldwide."

- Luffy Lv, CEO of Sonmol

Hence, after the pandemic, an evolution in clinical trials is inevitably necessary. Adopting patient-centric technologies will boost sponsorship of clinical trials. Sponsors should seek guidance from institutional review boards (IRBs). Now is the time to move from the health industry's conservative nature and other policies that need to be reviewed to save us from future embarrassments. The genie will not go back to the bottle. The time to resist change over improvements in vaccine developmental processes within the pharmaceutical industry is over. In recent years, the vaccine industry has the struggle to respond rapidly to epidemics.

Developing and commercializing vaccines for diseases such as Ebola, HINI, ZIKA, and SARS was incredibly challenging. The challenges stress the need for both development and manufacturing activities that could adapt to urgent demands. In the last decade, some biotech companies, governments, WHO, and research organizations have supported the development of platforms that could test epidemic pathogens associated with different viral families. Such endeavors are geared at speeding up the preliminary trial phases and could be used for clinical trials during subsequent outbreaks. The platforms of ideal interest to most sponsors are the RNA and DNA platforms. These platforms enable systemic processes that facilitate rapid testing of the vaccines.

Despite introducing such novel platforms, developing a vaccine for DARS-COV- 2 still poses challenges to developers and regulatory agencies. Pandemic experts continue to debate the best approaches that could ensure the most optimal immune responses. Experience tells us that the process for developing a vaccine is not only long but also expensive before a licensed vaccine gets to the market.

Therefore, instead of focusing on the linear pattern, which involves multiple checks before final production occurs, it is time to redesign a new vaccine approach for pandemics, including parallel execution of various steps within processes.

Such a design will speed the investigation process and reduce the financial burden that often weighs on sponsors and governments. For example, for preliminary clinical trials, both humans and animals could undergo parallel clinical test procedures. Such a design approach will facilitate rapid genetic sequencing and moving fast to the next stages.

Research and Development

Research and development are essential for potential growth and the maintenance of a relevant product in the market. The misconception is that R&D is the domain of high-tech technology companies or probably the major pharmaceutical companies. Much of their money is focused on designing new products and upgrading current designs in almost all existing consumer goods firms.

Besides, industries like pharmacies, high-tech goods, or software must invest substantially to improve product quality, while other companies may spend less than 5 percent of their research profits. The healthcare service sector needs to be revamped entirely to keep up with pandemics; better and more accessible testing facilities need to be introduced so that more people can be tested at a lower cost. In underdeveloped countries, people cannot afford to get tested and continue to live in their respective communities, causing the disease to spread in that environment.

The detection methods such as those of laser capture microdissection (L.C. M), confocal microscopy, proteomics, and In situ polymerase chain reaction assay needs extensive study and research so that modern techniques can allow for quicker results turnaround while reducing the risk of exposure to analysts, increasing sensitivity, safety, and preserving the strains without fragmentation.

More antiviral drugs need to be introduced, especially for the influenza strains currently present. Immune boosters, better medicines, and drugs, essential herbal medicine needs to be mass-produced and structured, so there is never an imbalance in the supply and demand chain. Most viruses transmit from animals. Animal cattle and husbandry should be improved. People should engage in better eating habits making sure their diets comprise of all essential nutrients. This would also help to improve their immunity. In developing countries, sanitation and waste management facilities need to be introduced. Sewerage facilities, which cause contamination of water, fruit and even affect marine wildlife, are inadequate.

Artificial Intelligence and other effective technologies should be incorporated in tracking the virus, keeping track of the mortality rate. Further Evaluations and research need to be carried out when developing medical devices to enhance accuracy and replace the old modules.

Moreover, studies and cross-examinations should be conducted in areas or regions that effectively fight the pandemics. Their techniques should become a part of the framework of these plans. Development should be enhanced so that biomedicine and other areas can adopt a multidisciplinary approach. This helps to navigate the initial stages of detecting the virus with greater ease to harness quicker results.

A few such approaches, for example, allowed the SARS COV 2 virus strain to be detected much faster than expected. A traditional culture formed from the strains of SARS was used. E.M. examinations were conducted on these clinical specimens and microbial tissue samples. The morphological coronavirus evidence was found with the anatomic and gene sequence localization through the detection process of both IHC, ISH, and PCR amplification. Thus, the etiological agent was found by comparing the new sequence with the old SARS stain. With this research, vaccines will be formed in a lesser amount of time, saving millions of lives. To prove the viability of a vaccine, quicker methods yielding similar results as that on mice should be researched so that the vaccine is again available for commercial use in a shorter period. Moreover, research should be done on the pathogenic, lethality, and spread so the virus can be contained as quickly as possible.

To increase health care capacity, health services need to be improved across all regions. This can occur only through the innovation and development of modern medicine to prevent potential pandemics. Development happens because of research, study, and exchange of databases. Hence, all countries should treat pandemics as a threat to global security and invest funds into research. Research in modern detection techniques, better immune supplements, better and more available antiviral drugs, and all drugs.

Test Laboratory Inefficiencies

The length of time used to evaluate diagnostics by federal agencies in many countries reduces the speed of valuable vaccines and other drugs to reach consumers. Most regulatory agencies presently have a framework that gives them much oversight and regulations on public health and private laboratories. An effort considered to slow down science advancements, especially during pandemic times. These controls prevent private laboratories from meeting the demand for reagents, especially with a slow supply chain. For example, if the tests go into the market on time, laboratory experts believe that the laboratory-developed test should not be considered a medical device despite regulatory agencies' oversight.

Despite the risk involved, such debates call for a level of reflexiveness on enforcing discretions with device manufacturers during pandemics. On the other hand, enhancing safety regulations and considering pre-certifications from other laboratories could expedite actions related to minimizing risks to patients. Despite all the governments' problems responding swiftly to COVID -19, it is undoubtedly true that solutions must relate to efficient leadership, regulation issues, and supply chain capabilities.

At the European level, the European medical association has harmonized a set of rules to guide investigators and sponsors of vaccine trials, such as blending data collection approaches and prioritizing a randomized approach in generating conclusive results. As governments scramble to contain the COVID-19 pandemic, providing medical care for affected patients has become a global challenge. The healthcare industry is struggling with inadequacy in PPE, overcrowding, and personnel deliverables. Like pharmaceutical companies, medical device manufacturers rely on both public and private laboratories for valuable clinical trial data.

To obtain market approval, most medical device manufacturers must deal with pre-post market clinical trials' headaches. In a pandemic that involves investigator-initiated studies (IIS), the outcome is sometimes unreliable because its efficiency depends on a broad consensus within a healthcare system. The medical device industry mostly relies on clinical trials mitigated by private sponsors. They depend on regulatory agency approvals, usually based on the investigated clinical performance's safety and reliability.

COVID- 19 Vaccine

Several approaches are being taken to develop the COVID 19 vaccine all around the world. An inactivated vaccine is when the virus strain is killed using a chemical and used for its development. Previously, vaccines for inactivated polio (shot), hepatitis A and rabies were made this way. Another approach includes a subunit vaccine. In this case, a virus is used to make the vaccine.

This is essential to provide immunity; it may be the spike protein for COVID- 19. Hepatitis and human papillomavirus vaccines were made this way. In a weakened live viral vaccine, the virus strain is made to grow in labs in a setup or cells, which is different from that of host cells; when the virus adapts to growing in this environment, it becomes less capable of thriving human host cells. When this is inserted in humans, it produces an immune response, which does not make the person sick but makes them immune.

Another approach involves a DNA vaccine, a gene that codes for the spike protein to COVID 19 are inserted in a circular DNA called plasmid to form a vaccine. An mRNA vaccine causes cells to make proteins for the virus. Once these proteins are made, the body stimulates an immune response to kill the proteins as antigens and develop immunity. A replicating viral vector vaccine, which was used to create a vaccine for Ebola, and a non-replicating viral vector vaccine are also in the works; however, it is a number game with vaccines.

Even after the vaccine is made, it will be needed to go under multiple testing rounds. Even then, no one can guarantee its effectiveness on everyone because of the coronavirus's changing and mutating nature. After a vaccine has passed these clinical trials, it will need to go under mass production before it is available for use locally. Even then, the age groups most at risk would get the vaccine first, so a long waiting period is still foreseen.

COVID-19 Vaccine from Moderna

The groundbreaking biotech company Moderna, Inc., announced that in phase three study for its COVID 19 vaccine candidate mRNA1273 trial met the statistical requirements of its candidate vaccine candidate COVID-19. Biotech company Moderna said that an early review of its phase 3 trial shows that its Covid-19 vaccine is 94.5 percent successful in preventing infection, giving hope for another breakthrough.

COVID-19 vaccine from Pfizer and BioNTech

In approximately 90 percent of participants in its Phase 3 clinical study, the COVID-19 vaccine being produced by Pfizer and BioNTech has proven effective for blocking the infection. It is based on data analyzed by an external, impartial committee responsible for monitoring the trial outcomes and only represents the trial's early results.

"Pfizer and BioNTech's vaccine candidate is an mRNA-based vaccine, a newer technology that many companies pursued COVID-19 in part because it offers some advantages in the pace of development and potential efficacy."

\- Darrell Etherington

Pfizer and Moderna plan to supply vaccines for hospitals and vaccination sites through private carriers, including UPS and FedEx. A vaccine candidate from Moderna remains stable at 2° to 8°C (36° to 46°F).

"We are pleased to submit these extended stability conditions for mRNA-1273 to regulators for approval. The ability to store our vaccine for up to 6 months at -20° C, including up to 30 days at normal refrigerator conditions after thawing, is an important development and would enable simpler distribution and more flexibility to facilitate wider-scale vaccination in the United States and other parts of the world."

\- Juan Andres, Chief Technical

Operations and Quality Officer at Moderna.

BioNTech and Pfizer candidates, BN1162b2 and BNT162b2, must be stored at a negative -94°F.These conditions could be satisfied in hospitals and laboratories and could be kept at these sites for immunization activities. One question could arise when distributing Covid-19 vaccines to hundreds of millions globally: Do we have enough freezers? ***Hence, a vaccine is never good enough until it turns to vaccination.***

Challenges of Manufacturing the Vaccine

Even after going through vaccine investigational regulatory procedures, bringing the product to the market needs expensive unconventional structures that could lead to manufacturing capacity. Unconventionally, developing novel technologies into platforms might involve surpassing licensing and other regulatory issues, but identifying and adapting transferred technology to the manufacturing process without understanding the vaccine candidate's viability is the biggest challenge.

Vaccine Distribution and Sensibilization

The production of COVID-19 vaccines is still a problem for biopharmaceutical companies. Given that one or more vaccines are licensed, several mechanisms to guide their ethical delivery remain debatable. However, even though intensive parallel efforts are ongoing to increase supply, there is no assurance that sufficient supply will be available to everyone in just a short time. The need for temperature-controlled storage of some vaccines to prevent infections to patients with underlying conditions is also troublesome.

There seems to be no globalized structure in place for large scale production and distribution. The World Health Organization (WHO) should ensure that the vaccines are not for highly developed nations but should legally be distributed to all affected countries. A global distribution system is necessary to execute such a magnanimous function. More so, it is time to take drastic measures to resolve logistics issues that have, for a long time, been affecting the healthcare industry. Below are four real solutions that can be used to mitigate similar issues:

Government Control

Governments should distribute initial vaccine supplies to states and territories. The authorities will then be responsible for targeting citizens and deciding which groups will be prioritized for the first doses. Some jurisdictions are required to participate in mass vaccination programs, including large retail pharmacies and hospitals.

Adequate funding for state and local governments

Government and health agencies need money and support to cope with this long-term pandemic. Specifically, for education and vaccination administration, additional hiring and training are required. Large-scale cooling is needed to store vaccines and technologies to monitor vaccines and maintain the inventory of vaccines. Many local health agencies are currently unable to handle the delivery of the vaccine at the required stage. Funds must be made available immediately to municipalities so that municipal authorities, local health workers, and policymakers can begin to incorporate specific infrastructure capabilities.

Collaboration with the private sector

Businesses in the private sector must step up to represent their neighborhoods, but it requires strong public and private collaborations. There are excellent guidelines for municipal courts, but the fact is that local health agencies do not have the money to enforce the recommendations. They cannot cool, transport, or technologies to ensure that community members are safely and efficiently vaccinated against coronavirus.

We need these corporations to step up, share their expertise with the communities around them, and participate in successful public-private collaborations to ensure that our communities can be effectively vaccinated. FedEx, DHL, Amazon, and more are required to increase the provision and distribution of cooling vaccines. We need Uber and Lyft to make sure that patients can enter vaccine hubs in difficult accessible regions. To step up and provide technology services that enable storage and sharing of data, we need Apple, Google, Oracle, IBM, and Epic, to help us understand who is completely immunized for successful tracking and monitoring.

Direct Supply to large companies

Millions of people need the vaccine. There could be little space for this kind of patient traffic in most of our local health centers. Big, local employers will play a significant role in ensuring the success of the last mile. Large businesses with several workers should be set up to vaccinate their staff. Companies with connections to broad areas or buildings can also use them as vaccine hubs. Vaccination centers should be built to support the community at places like arenas, theaters, and others that do not benefit from COVID-19 capacity.

CHAPTER SEVEN

Medical Devices Regulation
&
Harmonization Challenges

E ven if medical devices and other supplies can reach their destination in response to the crisis, many countries impose additional screening or quarantine measures for products from other countries. For example, ships that have previously visited China must also undergo improved inspection in Australia, Indonesia, South Korea, and many other countries. The FDA has suggested that this outbreak's consequences should not contribute to an increased risk to U.S. customers. Furthermore, no COVID-19 cases should be correlated in the United States with foreign manufactured products.

The U.S. Customs have targeted certain goods for U.S. imports that violate the laws of products controlled by the FDA. The Agency has not formally defined a program designed explicitly for COVID-19 unless it is willing to use its current authority to further sampling and screening or request further product information.

Regulatory Effects and Solutions for PPE Shortages

Unlike pharmaceutical companies, medical device manufacturers distributing products must not report any actual or potential supply chain shortages. Most regulatory bodies have sought to resolve possible shortages in the supply chain of medical devices. For instance, in an agency update, the FDA recognized that the outbreak COVID-19 is likely to impact the supply chain for medical supplies, including possible supply stops or shortages in the United States for essential medical supplies. FDA then started approving PPE using the EUA act, which gives the agency authority to approved specific devices during such outbreaks.

Following 63 manufacturers representing 72 facilities in China, the companies noticed that shipments were disrupted and could lead to potential shortages. While there are fewer national and international inspections, agencies are still able to track devices entering their borders with several tools, including import notices, enhanced sampling, and import screening, as well as data recovery before or after inspection, to keep track of medical devices that are being imported.

Imports from contract manufacturers in China, or even elsewhere, should also expect further sampling and import screening or request additional details on the federal agencies' goods. It is now more critical that all documentation is up to date to prevent unnecessary delays, given the likelihood of increased control on goods imported from China.

As medical device manufacturers deal with equipment, which is vital in the face of a global pandemic for various sub-populations, they may often be obliged to find new suppliers or even move production operations to new or different installations that suffer less from an outbreak. Although new suppliers or production facilities are expected to meet quality system regulations (QSR) requirements, businesses may be asked to apply specific measures in compliance with legal requirements.

Besides the relocation of production operations, specific life-support equipment may require submission and approval to join the market. Companies, therefore, need to understand how these changes can be made in times of crisis.

With this information, businesses should take steps to brace themselves for possible supply disturbances by recognizing that the agencies approving medical supplies, in some instances, with or without Emergency Use Authorization (EUA), have a vital role to play in the process.

COVID-19 adjusted Regulatory Pathway

The FDA has put in several efforts that enable fast regulatory processes for COVID-19 related medical devices. One such declaration is that it will be more comfortable and quicker to get regulatory approval for products that can help combat the COVID-19 pandemic. This declaration by the FDA is a sequel to the emergency authorization process (EUA). The EUA process now allows products that need pre-market notification to get approval for distribution within a few days rather than the usual long months before approval. This process is only applicable to products meant for a specific situation, especially emergencies that require urgent additional devices that improve the public's health protection. Compatible devices appropriate to this COVID-19 pandemic are oxygen ventilators and personal protective equipment like in-vitro diagnostics and mouth masks.

An EUA is open to products approved for a different use or not authorized for the USA. For example, the off-label use of the hydroxychloroquine drug, the manufacture of ventilators through medical device modification, and many newly developed in-vitro tests. The FDA also established a unique program whose sole purpose is to hasten the approval of COVID-19 treatments. This cleared two potential therapeutics for trial; so, it has already proven its worth. Relaxing requirements for specific product groups is another FDA COVID-19 regulatory measure.

Europe – Regulatory Response to COVID-19

It is essential to clarify the three classes of medical devices that the EU regulates. Part of class 1 devices are a subset of large devices which have become non-sterile and are not re-usable. Thus, these products are called "low-risk devices," and they can be self-certified. Therefore, there is a limited impact of the COVID-19 pandemic on this process. The whole group of class 2 and 3 devices and part of class 1 consist of other tools that must be marked for C.E. by a notified body. At the same time, the current situation gives rise to some complications.

These complications depend on the country that manufactures the medical device. European laws govern medical devices' approval, but the competent authorities at the national level control such regulations. Each European country controls its implementation and enforcement during this period. For example, authorities in the Netherlands and Ireland allow the commercial use of medical products once a healthcare institution indicates that they need the product, and no suitable alternative for such products are available.

Belgium, France, and a few other countries adjusted laws for the reuse of facial masks. At the European level, there has been an inauguration of the joint procurement agreement, which allows the joint purchase of personal protective equipment among member states. Other initiatives inaugurated the use of close contacts within the industry to increase production and improve medical equipment availability. Other efforts in place include controlling exports and promoting the free circulation of goods.

With these harmonized standards, companies can prove that their products or services comply with European legislation. Before this pandemic, companies would have to pay out hundreds of thousands of euros per standard. Apart from providing updated harmonized standards, class 1 medical devices' development and production are now more accessible through the E.U intervention.

Regulatory Oversight

Most regulatory agencies have expedited their decision-making process to meet with PPE demand during the COVID-19 pandemic. These regulatory agencies should not just focus on procedures that will accelerate application reviews or approvals but should implement measures leading to an oversight on supply chain safety. As standard protocols are maneuvered during a pandemic, the long and short-term impacts should be considered.

The regulatory agencies should embark on streamlining processes and procedures, incorporating telemedicine tools to ease patient and expert access to data during clinical trials and other investigational products as part of the monitoring process. Also, the introduction of virtual diagnostics and remote assessments should have a long term impact in expediting results during such periods, hoping that such suggestions will not minimize the value of advisory face-to-face committee meetings.

Harmonization of Medical Device Regulations

A robust and transparent regulatory framework, which is sustainable with fair market access internationally recognized by manufacturers, is needed to accompany the competitive market. A level of convergence should be encouraged in regulatory practices, so long as safety performance, effectiveness, and quality of the medical devices are assured. Such initiatives will lead to technological innovation and facilitate international trade.

Sometimes, it is difficult to evaluate the loss attained from unharmonized regulations because the consequences of too many regulations can only be measured through unnecessary hurdles and obstruction to productivity and economic performance.

Harmonization that increases economic demand creates significant incentives for businesses to become more profitable and sustainable. The variations and differences in safety regulations and risk management during new medical device development present many obstacles to introducing the product into the market. Regulatory bodies need to focus on timely, consistent, and effective pre-market and post-market regulations for medical devices that could be standardized.

A standardized regulation for medical devices reduces or eliminates unnecessary bottlenecks and requirements demanded by specific countries and brings transparency to manufacturers and marketers of these devices. Thus, enhancing cooperation amongst regulatory agencies of different countries and the requirements for each product lifecycle should be fully addressed. Such a move will reduce the complexities encountered in obtaining pre-market and post-market clearances and approvals for medical devices while promoting consumer confidence in many countries. Approval from relevant competent authorities worldwide shall be required when a new medical device is developed or enhanced before being marketed and distributed to the customer. The field of medical device legislation has changed significantly since the beginning of the 1980s.

More than 65 countries have regulations on medical devices enforced or will soon enforce medical devices' regulations. The word medical devices encompass everything from sophisticated computerized health equipment to basic wooden tongue depressors to the concept of suitable medical devices. Unlike pharmaceutical goods, it is not metabolic, immunological, or pharmacological that the primary mode of action is associated with a medical device on the body. There are various international medical device classification schemes in the world today.

With its companions, the World Health Organization works to harmonize medical devices' nomenclature, which dramatically impacts patient welfare. This is particularly necessary for recognizing accounts and recalls of adverse occurrences. A harmonized description has been suggested for medical devices by the Global Harmonization Task Force.

Medical device means such instruments, devices, implements, equipment, devices, implants, in-vitro calibrators or reagents, software or software, materials, or possibly another article intended by the manual manufacturer for disease diagnosis, surveillance, avoidance, alleviation, care, and monitoring.

Benefits of Harmonization During a Pandemic

If countries satisfy the required demand for their medical goods, they will make substantial profits. These gains would also allow them to fight any future pandemic. Harmonization helps the product to be standardized. It guarantees that the goods marketed or produced by rivals are of the highest quality.

With the growth of the market for a specific product, other competitors are being encouraged to work harder and create more inventions that further change the medical sciences. Product qualities do not only increase but cost also decreases considerably. These developments and innovations will lead to much more practical and intensive.

It was a worldwide situation as only a few pieces of equipment per thousand people was available. Had harmonization been achieved, ample test facilities would be open, including lower prices, to support developed and underdeveloped countries. In addition, the advancement and development in this technology will make it possible to deliver quicker diagnoses and outcomes to treat or isolate patients in a shorter period.

Harmonization also facilitates entrepreneurship and high-paid STEM jobs, contributing to medicines development and efficiently counter pandemics, such as COVID-19. Global R&D is now taking place, global clinical trials and laboratory sampling are taking place, various production sites, global product launches, and much more. Should this rivalry create better products that support us in pandemics?

In short, the harmonization of the regulation on medical devices is needed to minimize the time required for goods into the market, eliminating unjustified or incorrect country restrictions and making access accessible to patients clear and practicable. It also reduces the cost of the device by providing a clear global regulatory framework with specifications. It also cuts costs by removing obsolete machines that serve the same role and reduces the already limited financial and human capital.

Increasing collaboration through PMS procedures, joint audits, international standards adoption and use, the exchange of information on safety and security, the exchange of submission criteria, and more will enhance government performance. There will profuse assistance because harmonization and consumer access will be improved by implementing uniform specifications for all devices, reducing insecurity and burden to market clearance.

Finally and perhaps most significant of all, harmonization helps improve public health by providing a standard, well-known pre-market assessment and post-market monitoring control points, all of which will help ensure the consumer trust in the consistent performance of clinical safety tests.

Harmonizing regulations of medical devices have proven to be a significant step in the direction of medical innovation. These devices are predominantly used in the treatment of new pandemic viruses. However, some problems need to be addressed to ensure that these goods are more successful in innovation and accessibility to battle the many pandemic strains in the coming years. During the coronavirus pandemic, there would have been more medical supplies available internationally to provide the best care to all patients. There would not have been a lack of ventilators, detection devices, and even oximeters.

Harmonization Challenges in Asia

Asia is the leading medical device manufacturing continent. The medical device industry is increasingly shipping every day to the rest of the world. However, due to Asia's tremendous complexity, it is difficult to harmonize Asian legislation on medical devices.

These different factors vary from political and geological to social and cultural factors. As previously stated, these harmonization regulations allow for greater competition, lower costs, more innovation, and adaptive economies. It also gives the government tools to ensure that other policies, such as climate, health, quality, and safety, are respected.

However, policies vary from country to country, creating some disturbances in the process. Different parties have different priorities and do not consider medical equipment a priority. However, the situation is likely to change now that a global coronavirus recently infected the world. An enterprise that will benefit from harmonizing these regulations should also engage in open direct dialog with its ministers. In summary, there are cultural, political, linguistic, social, ethnic, and economic disparities. They also include philosophical differences, economics, infrastructure, skills, skilled workers, political interest, and regulation capacity.

Stakeholders cannot reach a consensus agreement on harmonization policies because the overall business configuration is different, and in product development, uncertainty prevails. Many countries have decades-long regulatory frameworks that are difficult to reform. As Asia is one of the biggest medical device manufacturers and markets, the situation needs to change as we start products that help us tackle epidemics. This situation could be mitigated through the implementation of a regulatory harmonization board system. This means that policies both at the political and local level are implemented. They set specific targets and infrastructure for the harmonization policies to be implemented. This regulatory framework is audited and checked regularly to ensure efficient product quality, protection, and expected targets. They should ensure that all these procedures are open, non-discriminatory, or affected by external powers on the international market.

Harmonized regulations should be regularly revised to reflect the changing policies and practices of the world. It will also help to remove rotational toon systems, which no longer offer advantages unless real evidence is available for their successful functioning. It will help to further improve the market and inspire stakeholders to spend more in their businesses to produce better-funded goods that are more capable of addressing modern challenges. To ensure they are up to date with the latest technologies, the FDA must upgrade Rating Systems.

These ranking systems identify various medical instruments, and better alternatives are needed for devices consistently reaching the lower ranks. The GHTF (Global Harmonization Task Force) must be stringent to ensure that all five of the GHTF policies instantly apply to stimulate a broader market with greater productivity and to allow for more framework excellence not only in Europe, Canada, Australia, Japan, and the United States but also in the rest of the world.

CHAPTER EIGHT

Integrating Pandemic Management

P andemic management has been referred to as the process of anticipating, responding, detecting, preparing, preventing, and controlling pandemics in order that deaths and adverse economic impacts are minimized. It is an all-embracing term that describes all that must be done before, during, and after pandemics. If the outbreak could not be prevented entirely, it involves preparedness so that there is a readiness to respond. Early detection through a sensitive surveillance system is necessary to know where and when the outbreak occurs to limit its spread.

Above all, a coordinated and rapid investigation is necessary to explain the outbreak and identify interventions that could be recommended as a reasonable response and applying appropriate control measures. Pandemics management would not be complete without analysis to determine what went right and wrong before and during the outbreak.

Although pandemic management requires knowledge of medical and public health, good management requires proper

128

coordination of all specialized areas involved in response activities. Information may be obtained rapidly from reference books as well as disease specialists. Experts in epidemiology, health education, clinical medicine, and laboratory medicine are required for a good pandemic response. The technical groups must be supported by public health authorities, management, and logistics experts. The epidemiologists are involved in outbreak investigation, surveillance, including contact tracing and follow-ups, and the prediction of pandemics.

The clinicians will be interested in managing the exposed, the ill, and the dead. Although laboratory testing might not be needed in all epidemics, the laboratory experts, if needed, are involved in specimen transportation, transfers, and diagnosis.
The need to prepare the general population and specific groups like the health workers is generally necessary during pandemics. The coordinating team consists of representatives of the technical subgroups, management personnel, and the logistics and is headed by the Commissioner for Health representative.

The staff provides the strategic directions for all the technical subgroups' responses plus liaises with the media and the political authority. The authority makes the decisions on infrastructure, etc., vaccinations, regulations, according to the recommendations from the coordinating group. The subgroups are expected to work in regular consultation with each other.

Integrated Disease Surveillance and Response (IDSR)

Disease prevention and preventative measures are successful if resources are dedicated to detecting a specific disease, collecting laboratory disease evidence, and utilizing district intervention thresholds. In the sense of enhanced public health monitoring and response in health faculties, national and districts, the World Health Organization (WHO) has correctly suggested an Integrated Disease Surveillance and Response (IDSR) strategy. The IDSR promotes fair use of resources through the incorporation and rationalization of day-to-day monitoring activities. Overview practices for various diseases have a similar function (detection, monitoring, appraisal and assessment, feedback, actions) and generally occur in the same structures, personnel, and processes. The IDSR refers to the One World Health point of view, which addresses humans, wildlife, household animals, and ecosystem health events. For example, 75% of new and recurrent human diseases (e.g., avian influenza, HIV / AIDS) have an animal origin.

We hope that these guidelines will give practitioners from various fields a better understanding of and help enhance cross-sectional integration with the structure, working, procedures, and processes that form the basis for disease surveillance, including human health outbreak investigation and response. When a pandemic virus has been detected, each region's immediate responsibility is to plan to avoid a pandemic and take institutionalized and sustainable measures in the fight against the epidemic.

However, a systematic approach should also be put in place at the earliest opportunity to mitigate the impact of the virus. For pandemics, which create new viruses as they spread simultaneously, preventive strategies are mostly universal. Depending on the epidemiology and pathogenesis of etiological viruses, specific adjustments are made to each process. The first step in integrating the preventive strategy is early detection of the virus.

It would be best if you then prepared the most comprehensively and substantially possible. Different strains of influenza and other viruses have pandemic potential but have not spread to the whole world.

The H5N1 strain rapidly infected and was often lethal in the bird population. This avian influenza may not have pandemic potential, but the coronavirus did the same but has now shown its potential to the world. COVID-19 has been an unbearable burden on all sectors, and thus a disease prevention policy must be adequately implemented in all the healthcare systems. Integration is now introduced to businesses.

Continuous planning must be developed, all industries' infrastructure optimized, and all useful implementation maintained at its heart. A new standard can be created, and vital tasks can be carried out even in a crisis state. The causes and effects of previous viruses, including recent coronaviruses, should be studied and preventive plans created. Another example is an extreme scarcity of antiviral agents. In at least 18 to 24 months, the vaccine will take effect. In addition, the vaccine can take months to be available in bulk for general use even after the vaccine has been produced. Recommendations from the World Health Organization's pandemic preparedness and prevention model would be the best way to plan now.

Tracking a Potential Virus

A six-phase process accurately assesses the threat of each existing strain of the virus, which a potential pandemic pose. There are three major branches of this process and six sub-branches. The first major branch is an inter-pandemic phase. In this phase, the virus has only shown animals' existence, and no human cases are reported. This further has two subcategories: low risk of human cases and the high risk of human cases. The next major branch is Pandemic Alert. This is when the new virus has caused human cases. This further comprises three subcategories: minimal human to human transmission, increased human to human transmission, and significant human to human transmission. As soon as there is a limited human transmission, that is an indication for one to bring in a prevention methodology or a risk mitigation plan.

The last major branch is that of a pandemic, and its subcategory is efficient, sustained, and continuous human to human transmissions with a high mortality rate. By phase 4, you need to start implementing these strategies, and by phase 5, the time for planning has passed. The need of the hour would be to carry out intensive execution of the plan.

Preparedness plans

All plans must start with education and awareness of the affected population. The virus should be addressed so that fear is not induced in the population, but they should be warned. Hygiene practices based on the study and research of the virus must be introduced, and people should be forced to implement them. Movement should be monitored at this point to make sure no one is traveling to risky areas. At the same time, isolation facilities and evacuation facilities should be in place as part of preparedness.

Since fear is as contagious as a virus, civic authorities have an undue burden to disrupt essential public services. This must be kept in mind when making contingency plans to minimize interruption in essential services. In any case, travel bans, and restrictions should be brought into place. People should be asked to avoid large gatherings depending on the transmission of the virus. Curfews and lockdowns might be implemented. In the recent outbreaks, many countries used a smart lockdown system where they screened the cities for most affected areas and locked them down to avoid the spread of the virus amongst communities.

A risk management team can help assess the economic losses caused by the shutting down of different services. Once these losses are estimated, ways to mitigate the losses must be brought in place.

Since pandemics are ever evolving, these policies should be flexible and adapt to changing circumstances. Encouraging tracking among people allows relaxation in taxes, allocates funds to help the most vulnerable, allows absentees, ease in work policies, and helps communities by engaging civil society and community leaders.

Donations and funding should be brought into place. Annual budget plans must be made in a way that reserves funds to help deal with outbreaks in case there are any. Infrastructure plans and civic amenities must be constructed to be well equipped and designed to deal with a pandemic.

Improvements - Public Health Sector

The public health sector does not only deal with the virus on the front line, but it also lays the groundwork for prevention. Therefore, research analysts, pathologists, microbiologists, virologists should be employed more in the coming years. They should be given incentives by the government, such as incremental pay or tax reduction.

In the coming years, the transmission of viruses from animals to humans has significantly increased. People from marginalized communities and communities that are most vulnerable to a pandemic's impacts should also be encouraged to partake in the public health sector by giving the scholarship to study and funds to research. Fellowship and learning opportunities should be increased. These people can then help save their communities. Health facilities should be overall improved. Common health issues should be put to bed once and for all. Health disparities should also be dealt with, so these facilities are again accessible to all-for example, opioid addictions, clean energy, environmental racism, homelessness, and more. Drugs and vaccine production should be increased, so their costs can be reduced.

What takes place in an integrated system?

1. The organization and streamlining of all surveillance operations. The resources are pooled to collect information from one central point on each floor, instead of using scarce resources to hold vertical operations apart.
2. Many operations are integrated into a single organized mission and use conventional monitoring positions, skills, resources, and target populations.

3. Acute flaccid paralysis (AFP) monitoring operations, for example, often include neonatal tetanus, measles, suspicious incidents, or other disease surveillance. Thus, health workers who visit healthcare centers to monitor AFP cases often search district and health records for information about some of the other diseases that are a priority in the region.

4. District level focus would be to incorporate supervisory functions. The district is also the leading health system with staff working on all public health levels, such as monitoring community-based health programs, mobilizing community action, encouraging federal funding, and accessing local resources to protect the district's health.

5. District, state and regional monitoring focal points collaborate with disease response committees at every level to organize and virtually explore the potential for pooling resources for unique public health response activities.

6. It focuses on developing a framework for surveillance of public health capable of detecting, responding to, and validating threats to non-communicable and transmissible diseases.

Systemic Integration

Refers to the harmonization of processes, software, types of data collection, standards, and case definitions for the prevention and maximization of effort among all prevention of diseases and management programs and stakeholders; only one data entry process for multiple diseases and frequent channels is used for countries with a standard reporting channel. A regular feedback newsletter is used, and additional online tools are exchanged, and supervisory models are incorporated.

The IDSR co-ordinates joint acts and surveillance operations almost daily (planning, tracking, execution, assessment) wherever possible and usefully.
Effective Coordination of the Health Management Information System services based on efficient information exchange, joint preparation, monitoring, and assessment ensure that stakeholders and policymakers at regional, national, and international levels are provided with reliable, appropriate, and consistent information and data.

The goal is to promote cooperation and coordination in a global, regional, and district multi-spectral, and multidisciplinary collaboration. The pandemic management system is responsible for organizing and monitoring activities in close cooperation or maybe in synergy with the pandemic response committee formed.

Objectives of IDSR
- Strengthen countries' capacity to conduct effective monitoring: staffing at all levels; creation and executing action plans; promotion and mobilizing capital.

137

- Integrate different control systems to allow more productive use of forms, materials, and personnel.

- Improving the use of information to identify shifting times to respond rapidly to recorded outbreaks and epidemics; tracking the impacts of interventions, including cases of fatality, spread, declining incidents, and promoting evidence-based response to public health events; developing health policy; planning; and managing Improving global monitoring flows. Reinforce lab expertise and interest in drug sensitivity and pathogens confirmation.

- Increase doctors' participation in the new control system.

- Emphasize community contribution to response and public health detection, including event-based response and surveillance under International Health Regulations (IHR) Causes epidemiological research to identify, track, and investigate public santé problems and introduce significant public health initiatives.

IDSR and IHR

- The main goal of the International Health Regulations (IHR), in a restricted way and unique to public health hazards and avoiding undue interference with international trade and trafficking, is to prevent, protect, track and resolve the global spread of disease.

- The IHR spectrum was expanded to all global public health crises, including cholera, plague, and yellow fever. This refers to disease sources, toxic weapons, hazardous materials, and tainted food. The IDSR offers the IHR to strengthen, at the district level, the overall national disease monitoring system, to ensure timely and continuous use and access to information for public health policy decision-making:
- Tracking, confirmation, question, reporting, and reply systems technology and services
- Man's Resource Seasoned
- Sensitization, assessment, action plan, execution, monitoring, and evaluation phase developed (sensitization)
- Generic assessment guides; production of action plans; technical guidance; training materials; IHR streamlined tools and standard operating procedures.

Prevention and Control Strategies

These guidelines presume that all health system levels are active in surveillance activities to identify and respond to priority diseases and conditions (though different levels do not perform the same functions).

These operations shall contain the following core functions:

Step 1: Identify incidents and instances. Use common case descriptions, define priority disorders, incidents, and conditions.

Phase 2: Report suspicious cases or incidents or symptoms to a higher level. Whether this is a pandemic-prone disease, or perhaps a Public Health Emergency of International Significance (PHEIC), or perhaps a disease targeted for eradication or elimination, respond immediately by testing the situation or perhaps by sending a comprehensive report. For incidents to be alerted under IHR, use the decision-making instrument (Annex 2 of IHR) to recognize any possible PHEICs.

Step 3: Analyze and interpret the results. Compile and evaluate data for patterns. Compare details with earlier periods and summarize the findings.

Step 4: Investigate and validate suspicious incidents, occurrences, or, likely, outbreaks. Please take steps to ensure that the case, epidemic, or possible occurrence is confirmed, including laboratory confirmation, whenever possible. Collect proof of what may have triggered an outbreak, or even an incident, and use it to choose effective prevention and control strategies.

Phase 5: Get packed. Take steps in advance of public health events or outbreaks so that teams can react relatively rapidly, and critical equipment and resources can be identified for immediate action —

step six Respond. Coordinate and mobilize staff and resources to respond effectively to public health.

Phase 6: Please provide input. Encourage future collaboration by engaging with the level of information given, recorded outbreaks, events, and cases on the investigation results and the response efforts' progress.

Phase 7: Assess and develop the commodity. Assess the importance of surveillance and response systems in timeliness, quality of information, thresholds, preparedness, overall performance, and case management. Take steps to resolve problems and make changes.

CHAPTER NINE

Demand Management Style

The economic impact of this pandemic is most visible in the consumer goods sector. Instead of house toilet paper and cleaning supplies, there have been images of empty shelves in news broadcasts and social media feeds. Consumers are making significant shifts to their shopping platforms. They wish to purchase items at an incredible scale and speed.

All consumer goods producers are making efforts to determine the magnitude of these changes in consumer behavior on their categories, channels, and brands during this crisis, and they are taking immediate actions. So, how can executives improve business performance?

The immediate reaction is for companies to maintain focus on business continuity to protect their employees and customers. Executives must optimize their business for the short-term while considering long-term measures and benefits. They must also discuss possible permanent shifts in consumer behavior after the pandemic so that they can make necessary adjustments to their business. This pivot involves new plans. In-crisis planning must be implemented within six weeks compared to normal annual planning processes, which may take between six to nine months.

Thus, consumer goods companies will have the speed and agility to navigate the crisis and emerge stronger. Consumer companies must launch a small and dedicated functional team with a committed leader to execute this 6-step plan.

Step 1: Size Revenue Exposure

Companies should diagnose their business goals by taking deep-dive category reviews across customers, geographies, brands, pack sizes, SKUs, and price tiers. By assessing the demand archetype applicable to each category, executives can:

- Compute possible revenue and profit pools.
- Understand the exposure levels of each category.
- Identify extra opportunities.

Such granular assessment not only supports prioritization by type but also specific brands, customers, and price tiers.

Step 2: Analyze Innovative Demand

Companies should project future demand once they have prioritized focus areas within a specific category.

Companies must be more sophisticated in their forecasting approach than in the past since it is now more important to understand both demand and actual consumption patterns that result in pantry loading.

Understanding the evolution of demand during and after the crisis at the most basic level involves using advanced analytic models with multiple sources of insights such as online search trends, social listening, primary consumer research, and point-of-sale data.

Also, you can gain greater clarity by asking the following questions:

- General: what is our perspective on the general virus containment and economic setting?
- Consumer behavior: what are the new priority consumer requirements? Is it health and safety attributes, value relevance, or higher e-commerce penetration?
- Categories: what demand models apply to individual categories, and are there any consequences?
- Channels and customers: what will be the effect of changing customer behavior on channel and store traffic?
- Portfolio and brand: In what areas will new consumer behaviors and preferences necessitate changes to the portfolio?
- Price tier: if consumers are unwilling to embrace changes to price, what is our alternative plan?

Step 3: Adapting the Marketing Plan

Executives can reflect changing consumption patterns and consumer sentiment by adapting their marketing plans rapidly. Reach, frequency, and Return on investments (ROI) should determine marketing spending. Executives must vary the tone of their creative marketing, mostly Ad copy and calls to action to flow with the current situation. Thus, the general consumer outlook will suit the stage of the pandemic response. Companies should also consider shifting to market spending in channels such as social and digital searches to reflect changing patterns and make it suitable for entertainment and media consumption. Real-time testing and measurement are the best ways to gauge these actions. Rapid testing should not be abandoned because we are experiencing an unprecedented crisis. The company can gather accurate data on the potency of current marketing efforts; then use the insights gained to adjust campaigns accordingly.

Step 4: Strengthening E-Commerce

Executives must implement any activity that can optimize the e-commerce channel quickly. Companies can form joint venture agreements with online retailers to augment existing capabilities, partner with online retailers, and boost customer collaboration. This collaboration might involve click-and-collect and skip-to-home offerings.

Demand (primarily, fast-selling SKUs) should determine the volume of products sent to e-commerce channels. Companies must perform demand forecasting anew every day. Thus, they can modify online inventory suitably, change logistics, and distribution channels to cater to online retailers' demands. Companies will invest in categories with a relatively stable order by performing a weekly review of all e-commerce promotions and advertising spending.

This review's side benefit is that they can hold off on discretionary categories of less importance to consumers. By having dedicated resources that manage SKU-level detail, product images, and merchandising tagging, companies can rapidly expand category management capabilities.

Step 5: Track the Three Ps(3Ps): Pricing, Promotions, And Portfolio

Companies should modify their promotional budgets and pricing plans to suit the expected demand curve throughout their portfolio. New promotion tactics must support products to lower the demand curves. Such tactics include combining high-demand and low-demand SKUs. Once expected, demand curves correspond with consumer priorities. Companies can add mix actions like executive support for higher-margin products, reduced promotions, and assortment adjustments. Thus, the adverse effects on other aspects of the portfolio will not be much. For affordability, companies can create consistent value-tier offerings simultaneously. By refreshing their revenue growth management analytics rapidly, companies can focus on factors affecting consumer buying behavior during the crisis. With this market analysis review, companies can make changes to their portfolio innovations. For instance, changes in consumer occasions and customer needs can determine when companies should reschedule their product launches.

Then, there should be a reallocation of resources, as necessary. The collective insights on the three Ps will help in planning the supply chain. Companies must make sure that portfolio planning, promotions, and the optimal price is a true reflection of the current realities with their supply chain. Companies can iterate plans over functions to understand the real financial impact and align supply-chain efficiencies with opportunities. They should act on these promotion and pricing insights over two-time horizons.

Companies should not make any price increments (even if it is a short-term increase) after the stay-at-home orders have been lifted. Customers will not forgive organizations that exploit the current situation for profits. Instead, executives must craft carefully targeted promotions to deepen connections with customers. They must re-evaluate planned pricing and promotion initiatives to suit significant changes in market structure.

Part of this step should involve the effect of specific brands or channels on consumers' shifting preferences.

Step 6: Partner with Consumers and Act

Through collaboration with customers to refine and deploy the revamped commercial plans, consumer goods companies can optimize the impact of their new plans. The essential aspects of this collaboration are flexibility and compression. Set the right tone by adjusting payment terms and making daily calls when necessary. There might be a need to implement various sales techniques, as well. Companies can improve virtual-selling techniques through the provision of extra support and technologies to their sales force. They should also reapportion field sales and brokerage resources to geographies, customers, and channels with high demand.

Companies that execute the 6-step plan will make significant progress when readjusting to the crisis and beyond. Before they can implement this 6-step plan, companies must adopt rapid, short bursts of work methodology. For optimal results, companies must establish a re-plan war room and create a fully committed and full-functional team that can meet virtually.

The team should use currently available data (regardless of the information) to make recommendations and decisions. Decision making will be rapid when executives can receive updates two times within a week. When companies can execute this plan successfully, they will have a clearer understanding of the market and even be ahead of the competition after the crisis. However, it will be too late for executives who decide to wait till after the pandemic to plan and act.

CHAPTER TEN

Hospital Capacity Management

The COVID-19 has exposed the unpreparedness of many governments and institutions in the world. Investing smartly will help mitigate future pandemics through the ability to detect and respond at record times. Despite the problem faced during prior outbreaks, the deficit in detecting and responding remains a growing problem as many nations struggle with testing, tracing, and capacity as a means of containing the infectious disease.

While most governments concentrate on solving the present crises, smart investments in COVID-19 response should be implemented towards other healthcare systems' preventive measures.

Building a healthcare infrastructure that does not rely on responding to an emergency, but a structure with all the tools needed to detect and respond to any crisis means our systems should meet crisis protocols, and healthcare workers are trained to meet demand. Furthermore, partnerships should be encouraged by the government in maintaining and sharing real-time information.

Whenever there is an outbreak, there is an immense burden on healthcare facilities. Naturally, most healthcare facilities are not designed to deal with an influx of patients, a topple over forces people to find refuge elsewhere, making them vulnerable to the impacts of a virus. Hospital capacities are tested and strained. There may be a lack of intensive care units, crucial medical equipment like ventilators, so we must learn how to ration them and make full use of available capacity.

During COVID– 19, Italy is a prime example of how limited hospital capacities can cause a massive blow to the whole country. Moreover, they can also cause surgery cancellations, extended stays at the hospital, and declining patient and staff satisfaction. Hospitals are forced to turn away patients, as it gets worse in the times of a pandemic. Due to more extended patient stays, staff must work overtime. Those who cannot find a bed at the hospital have to travel far and wide to get their required services.

While healthcare providers are purchasing, distributing, and utilizing high-cost services, there are still long lines in the emergency department with no free beddings. The best way to deal with this problem is through frequent interactions with health workers and timely addressing them. Patient safety and security must always be maintained. Creating capacity without new construction.

Improving Hospital Capacity

Most hospitals have probably existed for a certain period. Based on the history of the hospital, It is vital to check the sustained and efficient processes. Do they require more space? If yes, then build the required structure. Moreover, you need to assess the capacity available to you and patient demand. This way, you can rightly size the facility.

This allows space for a more massive patient influx of patients in case of such outbreaks. Homerooms, lunch areas, and cafes should be designed to ensure they can be effectively utilized without causing financial burdens to the hospital. Most hospitals keep closing and opening units temporarily, which also helps to avoid contamination through proper fumigation.

Information relating to improvements and data analysis should be stored to keep making informed decisions based on previous history. The data should also be available to the public and governing bodies, especially during a pandemic, controlling available space is available for patient transfers. A daily report of the hospital can also help when using data for resource allocation.

A 24/48-hour discharge plan should be maintained to see which bedding would be available. The timeline needs to be changed depending on the virus at hand and the recovery window. An annual capacity management assessment provides understanding on which decisions rendered good services and proposals for future demands.

Future resource allocation should be tracked. This will also help the hospital administration understand whether there is a persistent and recurring problem with capacity. All concerned departments must work cohesively to make sure there is always enough capacity.

The work synergy can be improved by deploying a logistics team, which is utterly concerned with dealing with this issue. The leaders must stay engaged with them throughout to make sure solutions are being produced, and thus favorable outcomes are being reached. The logistics team should reduce hospital diversions in accepting transfers whenever possible by creating space and facilities. This can only happen when there is organization-wide awareness about capacity management. A logistics team needs to be supported by a data analytics team.

Developing a Patient Dashboard

A team of analysts monitors the admission, recovery, and discharge of a patient using the patient dashboard. They also check when beds are available if they are being cleaned, replaced, etc. Transferred patients are also monitored. A transport notification system can help monitor the hospital traffic, where patients are moving, where the staff is moving, and more. Simply, moving a patient from

153

a bed unit to a waiting space while they are being discharged frees up crucial space.

This process needs to be streamlined. During pandemics, all patients who can be safely dealt with at home should be discharged to make space for acute conditions. Communication needs to be transparent among the hospital staff and other hospitals to ensure all patients are promptly dealt with, especially in times of a pandemic.

Moreover, comprehending what is being said is equally important too. Any miscommunication can cause a huge upset. These would also ensure the safe and timely transfer of patients from one department of care to another. Hospitalists and strategists can help place policies that can help reduce the effects of an increased patient burden while maintaining and optimizing patient care levels.

To manage patient flow, make sure that hospital beds are being utilized by patients who need them. Increase emergency care timing hours, this way, people with minor symptoms can be dealt with without delays; hence their situation will not escalate, and they would not need to be propped up on a bed.

Creating Hospital Extensions

Since a pandemic is probably underway, all other non-emergency surgeries must have been halted. This opens space in the post-surgery unit, use this space and turn it into an intensive care unit to deal with the patient surge. Rehab, psych, and other wards can also be used for the same purpose. Lobbies, cafeterias, waiting rooms, and hallways are all referred to as flat spaces, increasing the hospital's capacity.

You can start adding one or even two beds to private rooms since they have more significant spaces and must be used for the influx. To deal with patients' surge, spaces will need to be freed up and converted into medical centers rapidly to meet the demand. In most countries, football fields, cricket stadiums, and even hotels have been made into pandemic response centers.

These actions allow for isolation and reduce the contact from patients to the medical workforce, like in places where the hospitals have gotten too crowded. These potential spaces can be found in the community as well. They can be anything from marriage halls to college dorms and more. These spaces will also prove crucial since they will also be needed to set up testing facilities, isolation wards, quarantine wards, and treatment areas.

Hiring additional Workforce

To improve healthcare capacity, you will need more staffs. Additional staffs would be required to not only treat and care for the patients but also test them, isolate them, quarantine them, research for vaccines, study and analyze the virus strain, and even more cleaning staff to carry out daily fumigation to prevent infections in the hospitals.

Pharmaceutical staff would be needed to meet up with the demand too. All of this would require hospitals and establishments to hire and allocate additional staff. This can happen quickly if the government foresees a pandemic and provides funding to related departments to devise a cure. At the same time, scholarships and financial aid can be provided to prospective medical students to aid in the process. Drugstore vendors can be given tax relaxation or duty-free imports to make medicines readily accessible to the general population. Moreover, I.T technicians would also be needed to run data analysis and a logistics team to assist the hospital staff.

More nurses would also be needed as secondary caregivers. Thus, local people should be asked to volunteer and donate as much as possible to the organization. In many underdeveloped and developing countries, local businessmen were given incentives to produce masks, gloves, and PPE suits during the COVID 19 pandemic. Moreover, in these countries, students in their last year of medical school were also employed to meet additional demand.

The local population was asked to become part of a volunteer task force required to guard isolation and quarantine centers or track the virus's spread so the chain could be broken. In wealthier countries where the medical health facilities are better, the death toll reached an all-time high, shocking. A doctor was available for every 250 patients, but still, so many deaths occurred.

In underdeveloped countries where there is one doctor for every 1000 patients, the situation is drastically worse. There are three ventilators available for 1 Million people. Therefore, there is a need to harmonize medical devices' regulations to increase these devices' production and quality.

A pre-COVID-19 examination of the world health security index showed that no country was ready for a pandemic, and so the strategy 'do what it takes' was devised. As a result, the world's 85 poorest countries were given a sum of 160 USD billion to save the lives of around 3.7 billion people. Moreover, their debts were cancelled. But did that help?

Since the pandemic is global, doctors and medical health specialists also travel among countries to assist countries on the worst receiving end. In developing and underdeveloped nations, lockdowns cannot be imposed because most of the population comprises daily wagers; people who earned daily, and if a lockdown were imposed, they would have no mode of earnings would die out of lack of food and water. Similarly, people living in these countries lack essential health and water facilities, which gives rise to tons of other medical emergencies like dysentery, cholera, typhoid, malaria, and more.

They also live in close communities, so if one person contracted the virus, it was impossible for them not to transmit it to someone else. In a convention in May, these countries were given hefty donations, doctors and medical supplies were sent to equip them and save them from mass deaths.

Initially, this felt inevitable, with hospitals lining up with dead bodies and doctors being forced to decide whom to save and who not to save, but with the help of the entire world, the situation did get significantly better.

To avoid the COVID-19 pandemic situation in the future, underdeveloped countries' health profile index needs to be collectively worked over by the strongest nations. Sanitary and sewage facilities must be developed in such areas. Doctors should be given incentives to volunteer in underdeveloped areas. Funding and aid should be increased in such countries.

CHAPTER ELEVEN

Reimagining Healthcare for Pandemics

While it is great to have a COVID-19 vaccine, going disease by disease, vaccine by vaccine, specific treatments by specific treatments will not solve our larger problem for emerging epidemics, and there are several reasons why that is inadequate. First, if the vaccine is available, we can have the biomedical technology, but without the infrastructure and the resources needed, you cannot deliver amazingly effective medicines and vaccines.

There is an inadequate structure to ensure that we can get these technologies to the people who need them most. Also, there must be an integration of scientific solutions with social policies. The term that gets thrown around a lot right now is infrastructure and capacity. Capacity and infrastructure are rarely solved in a moment of crisis. They require investments, and one cannot build the bridge or fix the bridge in the middle of an accident. That analogy is vital in healthcare because we often focus on infrastructure in the middle of a crisis, where everyone is just trying to put out the crisis.

We know that infections have always been present and have always been a crucial element of global health. Nevertheless, a group of infectious disease experts, public health officials, vaccine scientists came together in the early '90s and produced a report that disclosed emerging new infections could just have tragic implications for global health in the United States and around the world. They were also of the notion that there could be infectious agents that we have not identified, which will pose significant crucial risks and what should be done.

We could have anticipated better vaccine research on some known agents, public health infrastructural and surveillance mechanisms, early intervention in the face of certain infections that could quickly spread, and better public health education. COVID-19 exposed significant problems with our public health infrastructure.

One brutal irony of COVID-19 is that it exposed that we have not maintained an up-to-date, rational, scientific, public health infrastructure.

Remembering the Lessons

Why is it that we do not learn our lessons from the previous pandemic? When things have persisted, and we know that we are in it for a longer haul, we tend to think more longitudinally across disciplines and approaches. However, when we assume something is an immediate crisis that might resolve itself for reasons, we do not entirely understand that we sort of fall back to the status quo. We need to think more clearly about generalizable principles of public health, prevention, education, communication, investment in science that will cut across disease and epidemics, as well as access to care.

Such endeavors require more systematic thinking because there were certain things that we knew before the pandemic. Thus, having sufficient personal protective equipment can be used across many different infections and create much better survival. We do not want to make the COVID-19 outbreak last any longer.
There are so many powerful and admittedly tragic elements to COVID-19 that need to be enforced more profoundly, including policy and practice. There should be a structure to rapidly deploy public health experts and healthcare providers on the ground to places where epidemics might break out.

Apart from the knowledge gained, what we will do at the next pandemic outbreak? We need to have greater flexibility and understand the possibility that certain types of interventions are not generalizable.

Sometimes, an epidemic could create opportunities where we begin to build proper health infrastructure. Thus, there will always be the availability of institutions, structures, and human capacities for quick notification, better communication, and intelligent deployment of resources.

The laboratories must be integrated into a broader analysis of the determinants of diseases. Those are the places where we fail, and we often fail because everyone says, *"Well, that is hard, and I am not going to think about that now. I will think about it later."* One of the things that history teaches us is that we must think about the long term. When we do that, we can plan and impact the future.

However, when we are thinking about a short-term crisis and cannot project that into a set of strategies that might take 10 to 20 years to implement, we will likely put those things off our immediate needs and concerns.

The truth is that it is challenging to balance the public policy and political perspectives. However, if we want to resolve global health issues that affect every one of us, we must start thinking or reimagining how our healthcare systems could effectively be used to manage pandemics.

Managers have always considered OEM sales as one of their favorite indicators to measure success. In this crucial time, managers must look beyond such measures and concentrate on the chain of reactions that encourage the timely delivery of medical supplies to hospitals, clinics, and healthcare professionals.

The COVID -19 provides a reason for OEMs to evaluate their inventories because the previous epidemics (Zika, HIV, Ebola, Malaria) of the 20th century were limited to specific areas and specific populations; things change over time. Hence, OEMs must consider suppliers not only on regularity but also on the reliability of supplies that best suit other crises or global pandemics. Suppliers that prove readiness to adapt to disasters should be rewarded in the future.

Lessons for Everyone

This pandemic exposes the fact that we have not developed the mechanisms for epidemiological surveillance that would be incredibly helpful and protective. There is no sure access to the healthcare system crucial than public health emergencies. We have a set of state-oriented programs, and there is high variability in terms of the state's apparatus and effectiveness in dealing with public health emergencies, crises, and epidemics.

More must be done in terms of surveilling people coming from places that were being most affected by the epidemic. The uncertainty and the processes of deciding how to manage air traffic are gigantic issues. Currently, there is minimal global governance over international air travel. Nevertheless, there is no rational set of policies for the healthcare industry with significant economic impacts worldwide. Unfortunately, these episodes often fail to generate thinking, process, and policy that would be good for everyone.

Healthcare Lean Six Sigma "Adopting JIT and JIC"

During a pandemic, many employees of businesses could work remotely from home. Meetings are conducted using tools like zoom, facetime, and skype. The inability of employees to physically interact still poses a problem to companies. Lean six sigma practitioners should think of creating visibility in projects by integrating visual management and process mapping tools that will be used to develop workflow and workstreams that can enable live monitoring of projects with assigned timelines for completing each task.

Using the lean supply chain method enables thorough planning, visibility, stability, reliability, and a collaborative network that provides a first-class operational-feedback loop. Such initiatives trigger a pull, which sets the pace for operations to deliver goods to the customer at a lower cost. Instead of maintaining the "Just in

Time (JIT)" strategy of Toyota. What the COVID-19 outbreak has taught us is to consider introducing the 'just in case' approach.

If most companies adopted the "Just in Case (JIC)' approach, we might have avoided PPE's embarrassment and other product shortages required to fight the Coronavirus. I do not buy the argument that a lean supply chain is a process of minimizing inventory. Instead, the thin supply chain should be considered as a method of inventory optimization. At what level should the stock be optimized? That is a debate between warehouse managers and logistics experts should be welcoming.

Private enterprises optimize their inventories at levels that relate mostly to one stocking level called the cycle stock. Their lists can only meet average demand, and the optimization involves three stocking levels. The stocking levels include cycle stock, buffer stock, and safety stock. The buffer stock levels that protect common cause variations in demand and safety stock protect against extraordinary incidents and crises.

Hence, the last two variables should be considered as 'just in case' models. Because most private enterprises cannot sustain all three inventory levels, the government agencies must team up with corporations to prepare for emergencies like COVID-19. There is no doubt that we have seen progress both through the international health regulatory body and government agencies.

Despite these improvements, some significant challenges and gaps prevent the smooth preparedness for global pandemics. COVID-19 has exposed gaps related to worldwide coordination and mobilization of resources. A framework to ensure the timely detection of the virus, tracing and quarantine procedures are still lacking.

"And while we have talked about the operational disruptions and how we are tackling those, I've been pleased at how our teams have responded to the calls for support from our clients as they rapidly design and procure solutions to address the pandemic. Our ability to quickly pivot has underscored the resilience of our business model and our position as a trusted partner to governments worldwide"-Bruce Caswell, President and CEO Maximus

Use of Artificial Intelligence and Modern Technology

Modern technology and databases can help make the fight against pandemics an easy one. Applications and software can be introduced which monitor the spread of viruses so areas can undergo a phase or smart lockdown.

Access should be provided, so managers could monitor bed capacity in different hospitals. They can record and store patients' previous clinical data to be effectively treated for the virus, given that the virus may exacerbate other underlying health issues. I.T workers can also provide online service to people in remote places so that contact and travelling are reduced during the times of a pandemic.

These services can be anything from diagnosis to counselling for people suffering from mental health issues.

Moreover, mobile clinic services should be introduced for rural and underdeveloped areas. This could work exceptionally well for under-developed countries where resources are not available to build better clinics. Alternatively, only a few doctors exist for most populated cities. This could reduce the commute distance for people.

Funding to Countries at the Forefront

You can have an excellent prevention plan in place, you are prepared to deal with it all, but since a tonne of moving factors is involved in a pandemic, it is nearly impossible to stop an outbreak. You can reduce its impact by localizing it, but it will spread, so the best way to prevent it is by fighting it at its root. As soon as you detect a virus spreading in a region, send your medical specialists and analysts to collect samples and help the general population. Send them funds to fight the virus and conduct research to find vaccines along with their professionals.

A pandemic cannot be stopped anywhere until it is stopped everywhere. All countries, which are part of the United Nations and WHO, must donate funds and make sure impoverished countries

167

have medical equipment, surveillance networks, isolation facilities, laboratories and testing facilities, supplies including medicines, a healthy workforce of doctors and nurses, and more. Global Health Security agenda should be updated so that all countries meet the WHO's health guidelines, so all outbreaks are effectively mitigated as soon as they start.

"The response to the COVID-19 pandemic has shown us some of the best of humanity: pathbreaking innovation, heroic acts by frontline workers, and ordinary people doing the best they can for their families, neighbors, and communities."

- Bill Gates Bill, Co-chair, Bill & Melinda Gates Foundation

It is a costly idea with an unpredictable wage for retooling a manufacturing plant to make medical devices because of emergency needs. It is also harder to ask since suppliers are not charged before the goods are shipped. They can also never see revenue before the full costs of developing and recruiting skilled employees have been incurred. The federal government should give guaranteed credit to businesses wishing to start the N95 enterprise as a more acceptable alternative. More significantly, these companies must be guaranteed by the government to purchase most of the masks slightly above the regular cost.

An estimation of the number of masks necessary and the time required should be made for optimal performance. The government would then ensure that more masks are purchased. The country will thus recover the overwhelming PPE demand as predicted. However, if supply goes far beyond demand, the enterprises cannot generate the PPE at a loss.

The surplus can be added or aid countries with little income who cannot generate what they need. The Swab, Hand sanitizers, and other essential products, which are not available, should apply the same strategy. This act is not only an actual business model but a goodwill model. The government would help manage purchasing contracts for goods with low stocks at high prices. Meanwhile, regulatory authorities need to change risk evaluations to meet the urgency of the crisis.

Coordinative Efforts by Governments

In addition to having a supply-enhanced environment, governments need to ensure that the affected areas receive the required equipment at any time. Resources should be allocated according to needs. It is highly likely that COVID-19 will spread simultaneously in all parts of the world and that there will be a chance to organize resources to fill the gaps. For example, other communities with few cases can share supplies with New York City because its COVID-19 cases are significantly increasing than other states. When the surge subsides, New York will move its equipment to a new community with growing cases. To ensure that both supply and demand are in line, the availability of the expected equipment needs can be tracked in real-time through collaboration with I.T. companies.

Patients would be protected by supplying essential equipment for hospitals and ICUs around the world. The European Committee aims to prevent shortages in personal safety devices, medical equipment, and medicines through the European Medicines Agency.

The committee has also given a guideline on adequate and rapid response to pandemics for notified bodies and competent national authorities. These necessary steps have improved the ability to move sufficient medical equipment to facilities. Examples: Ford and General Electric work together to create ventilators. As part of its fleet of household appliances, Dyson currently sells hospital fans. 3D enterprises and other smaller companies have open-sourced designs to speed up face shield production.

Engaging Underdeveloped Countries

During my philanthropic work at the time of Ebola outbreak in West Africa, I considered pandemics to be another sign of human connection within a world that remains more interconnected than the last century. Instead of considering SARS-CoV-2 a "foreign virus," I believe it is a global responsibility, which deserves a humane response. We may not have had the ability to drastically stop the pandemic but still have a chance because the established areas of responsibility remain the same.

Poor countries are facing significant economic difficulties. The pandemic made a terrible situation even worse. For years, these countries have been calling for funding to construct economic development infrastructure. The companies are relatively small in these countries and do not have access to financing. The effect of COVID-19 on countries should not be underestimated. However, I think a glimmer of hope remains. The situation today provides an opportunity to focus on what can be done to make these countries more resilient.

These countries and companies have the possibility to start innovating, as SMEs are typically flexible and capable of adapting to changes. For example, companies should be able innovate existing value chains and survive through e-commerce. There is an opportunity to focus on how we can build more robust value chains for future pandemics. We must pursue more long-term, cheaper and environmentally sustainable production options.

" We know the African energy sector can make an incredible rebound and that the opportunities for investment and growth will be exponential, but the energy industry must first be reshaped

for a post-COVID-19 comeback"-NJ Ayuk, Chairman African Energy Chamber

There is an overall lack of basic health necessities in such areas, causing many deaths in a short period. Cumulative effects include altered health-seeking behavior and postponement of treatment. Doctors from other countries should be encouraged and motivated to help all those who suffer from a pandemic's impact, be it in any country. Marginalized communities should be given financial support during such times to make sure they can afford to have the same level of care.

Dispensaries and other disposal clinics should be set up so that some level of medical care is available. The usage of herbal medicine must be prevented unless advised by a professional. Self-medication and addictions pose yet another threat towards better medical practices and thus should be deterred.

Millions of people are immigrating to other developed areas during this coronavirus pandemic crisis, this has proven to be fatal as the transmission increases. People were asked to flee back to their countries of origin, which they could not do since their countries' situation was worse. Most of these people are usually fleeing because of gang crimes, terrorism, genocides, and more. The UNO needs to investigate refugees' security and health and of under-develop countries; otherwise, pandemics will continue to rage.

WHO Needs to Be More Authoritative

Compliance is always a problem with international law, especially in the health industry. The world trade organization should allow states to impose trade sanctions and adjudicate problems through its judicial-like body. Then, the WHO does the same by holding states to account, but they have not. Though the WHO and other organizations will never have full command and control of the global health sector, there are ways in which they can enhance compliance.

The director-general and member states need to say, *"There is our requirement, and here is the funding for that requirement because that has not happened. We will then subject the sector to rigorous external assessments and evaluations that you must strongly adhere to; we will stress-test you. We are going to put you through paces and make it public. Hence, transparency becomes a major form of accountability."*

That would go a long way. However, it has not happened. Nevertheless, beyond that, we could have civil society shadow reporting like the humanitarian and human rights concerns. You can have noticeably clear targets and benchmarks that require monitoring and reporting.

Whether it is because we do not have the money, the political will, or just a dying culture, we cannot let national governments off the hook. It is primarily a national problem and a governmental problem. So, we need to hold governments to account.

Recommendations for outbreak control were supposed to have been implemented earlier. Such recommendations include setting up isolation centers, providing vast amounts of personal protective equipment, and travel restrictions. WHO could have used the bully pulpit. The director-general should have stated publicly and declare the disease as a pandemic and disclose other information earlier than they did. The WHO should have had many intense negotiations with governments and others to discuss what is acceptable.

How Should WHO respond?

It starts with the WHO's reformation, makes it transparent, holds it accountable, and has civil society involved in its governance structures, ensuring that the Director-general is a strong leader with political backing and stature. We need to make WHO effective, transparent, accountable. Then, we need to develop health systems and core capacities. There must be an exact mechanism to partner with countries to put in the money, close those capacity gaps, and assess externally and stress-test.

Also, there is the vital role of health workers. Some of the West African countries affected by the pandemic. They have some of the lowest proportion of health workers to patients globally - way below the bare minimum of WHO requirements. They even lost many of these workers - most left their job or died during the outbreak. - it was terrible. Also, there must be the availability of a well-trained international health workforce that is well-funded, accountable, and well-prepared to help in an emergency.

We must then ensure that we have controlled infection because it is the health workers at the most significant risk, and patients are also at risk. Hence, healthcare settings need to be safe, humane, and useful places to prevent them from leaving in droves. During this COVID-19 pandemic, more people have died unnecessarily due to malaria, tuberculosis, unsafe childbirth. They died because the health system collapsed.

Investments needed

There are so many things to be done. How do you identify the priorities and do them, right? That kind of pragmatism is necessary to slow, then halt an epidemic like this and save lives. At the same time, we are now in a situation where one of the chief tasks before us is to build a healthcare delivery system that can deliver on disease control and surveillance control so that infectious disease doctors will use it. Also, we need a way to provide adequate care for infected persons and address trust issues.

However, the number one task before us is to help divert enough resources into strengthening the health system, including the staff, tools, space, and systems. There is an urgent need to address the human resources for a health crisis. While that has been there for a long time, it is worse now, and it is not going to be addressed by physicians or nurses only. We need community health workers, managers, physicians, and nurses. You cannot have a healthcare system without people who deliver healthcare.

Apart from COVID-19, there is a spike in maternal mortality, outbreaks of pertussis, measles, and other health challenges. Hence, building an entire health system is an absolute necessity. However, there is not much evidence of significant investments in healthcare delivery systems. What has happened is another wake-up call that we need to figure out different ways of organizing R&D.

Furthermore, we need to figure out ways of not only addressing the problem of neglected diseases, such as Ebola and diseases that have high pandemic risk and are extremely lethal, are hugely risky for other reasons, or have never even emerged before, such as COVID-19.

We need to figure out a way to do R&D for new emerging infectious diseases. There are many categories of diseases for which the standard industry-driven R & D model will not work because we do not have the right incentives or rules.

So far, what we have seen during the COVID-19 outbreak has been encouraging in some ways. For example, the WHO played an essential role in bringing together major players involved in R&D, including research funders, the industry, and groups on the ground like MSF, who put in place clinical trials quickly.

Thus, there has been the mobilization of clinical trial efforts in record time. Unfortunately, we still do not have an approved vaccine. We still do not have any approved drugs. We do not know how well convalescent plasma will work for patients since we have not used it; Nevertheless, clinical studies are needed to prove its safety and effectiveness.

This is not just about R&D in terms of products, but broader research questions regarding intervention strategies. We still do not know much about the use of Remdesivir or convalescent plasma. There are many open research questions, but these highlights need us to organize ourselves better ahead of an emergency.

Then, figure out the technology, products, and some more operational questions such as, how do you organize a system to put the investments in place and generate sufficient information that ensures that the knowledge is shared more rapidly during an outbreak?

Also, there should be clear rules for researchers, especially in terms of data sharing. There should be explicit norms and expectations that, in an emergency, scientists would share their data for the greater, broader public interest of improving, understanding, and counteracting a similar outbreak soon. Currently, there are no norms or rules like that.

Stopping Climate Change Driven Diseases

Most zoonotic diseases, including MERS, SARS, and SARS COV 2, if not all, share one root cause, and that is climate change. Climate change has caused the temperatures to fluctuate wildly and laid great stress on individual immune systems. Moreover, deforestation and urbanization have caused migration among animals. Encroachment into wildlife and the destruction of indigenous lands and communities have caused an imbalance in the ecosystem.

Climate change needs to be recognized right now and should be fought globally. Funds must be allocated to combat climate change and effectively change policies to reduce our carbon footprint and make the world practices more eco-friendly. Burning the Amazon, illegal logging, uptake of indigenous land should be banned. Wildlife trade should be banned as well. To integrate a well-thought-out prevention plan into the existing manuscript of a region is the duty of the policymakers and leaders of that region.

The local population must force them to bring in such action plans and clearly define roles and responsibilities. With innovation in Artificial intelligence and other detection practices, such viruses should be predicted long before any outbreak so that a prevention plan is already drawn up. Disease and vector surveillance departments should be funded along with research and development, institution and capacity building, health, education, communication, and media sector.

All comprehensive health programs should include preventative, rehabilitative, promotive, and curative measures. Preparedness should always be ensured. Investment in research and development is vital to make sure your preventative strategy is comprehensive and flexible. For the local population, preventative measures would include but not be limited to building a stronger immunity, whether by taking supplements or taking a strict diet to make sure all your needs are met according to your gender, age, and nature.

They should also be prepared to treat themselves at home because there is a breakage in the supply and demand chain during a pandemic. Isolation and sick rooms should be created in your household space for such situations. You should also investigate trying herbal and natural Ayurveda medicines. Lastly, pandemics come from psychological effects, including depression, over thinking, fear, and more. So, help your friends, family, and loved ones adjust to the new normal.

CHAPTER TWELVE

Conclusions

E pidemic preparedness constitutes all the activities that need to be undertaken at all levels to respond appropriately to disease outbreaks. Pandemic preparedness elements will include the routine surveillance system that can detect outbreaks when it occurs and ensure resources to confirm, investigate, and respond to outbreaks are available. During the pandemic preparedness period, buffer stocks of drugs, equipment, materials, and supplies are enhanced.

Med-Chains directly focuses on helping health experts identify, prioritize, and successfully tackle quality improvement in healthcare. With the proper investigation and analysis, healthcare providers and improvement teams can completely transform healthcare, improving the quality of care delivered to patients.

A roadmap to use best practices, adoption, and analytics in concert to drive outcomes improvement is the main objective. A debate on integration and collaboration relating to disease surveillance, outbreak investigation, and response activities of professionals in various fields reinforces and enhances intersectional links to enable efficient use of limited resources, prompt and effective utilization of different sectors' capacities to improve disease surveillance. One of the most frustrating things is that health workers on the front line are begging for more masks, protective coats, test sets, fans, and intensive unit beds as we struggle to solve the Covid-19 pandemic.

Avoiding Past Mistakes

The crisis is based on just-in-time inventory principles. 'inventory is waste' is a discipline and a mantra derived from Toyota's production system. This concept has become popular in supply chain and corporate productivity and is embraced by industries worldwide.

The JIT concept demands that companies and their providers retain lean stocks and close relations with customers. The concept decreases the costs of the supply chain and production.

It also decreases reaction times in the supply chain, enabling businesses to adapt to shifts in the market more quickly. The movement started with car manufacturing, where systems that brought together numerous components on one assembly site were ripe for efficiency efforts. All kinds of industries have applied these principles, including the healthcare industry. When hospital JIT supply chains work as advertised, the savings in those expensive, high-stakes systems can be significant.

However, supply chains built on accurate and timely deliveries are vulnerable to unexpected and large-scale disruptions. The consequences can become acute when supply is unavailable when demand peaks. This is one of the main reasons why the pandemic supply chains in healthcare are paralyzed. The outbreak that started in a single region of China entered a global crisis as demand for medical equipment outstripped supply due to the rapid spread of infections worldwide.

Due to colossal leadership failures in many, healthcare providers and hospitals have competed for personal protective equipment and other medical devices. That has raised supplier prices and introduced unpredictability in procurement processes. Scrupulous players began selling fictitious and below standard equipment, as did several more parts and material shortages.

JIT networks and storages are incapable of meeting the challenge; therefore, medical supply chains should be more equipped for these outbreaks, like just-in-case storage. However, it is too much to forgive the benefits of just-in-time activities. Organizations that depend on massive stocks will not cope with slender facilities for hospitals. Instead, a required inventory of emergencies should be available. One way is to manage medical equipment inventory, just as banks treat the Federal Reserve.

Financial institutions must maintain absolute reserves and undergo a financial stress test. Although a higher inventory may be needed in hospitals and health clinics by licenses and regulations, this has not proven to be enough and adequate. Instead, we need to maintain a robust central inventory of healthcare supplies at different locations worldwide to complement each hospital's inventory.

The USA built its Strategic Petroleum Reserve (SPR) as a net oil importer. The SPR is not used to modulate daily oil price fluctuations; however, it can be triggered upon the President's approval if significant shortages occur. Similarly, in emergencies, America can store personal protective devices, fans, and other essential gears. Yes, the availability of medical supplies in the United States is available, but it was not enough for such a pandemic. A much more extensive and more professionally managed inventory of emergencies is needed.

They should also subsidize the production capacity needed to maintain the stocks of essential health supplies, just as the Pentagon supports US weapons producers. The pandemic of Covid-19 tells us that the state must do the same for vital medical supplies. To keep inventory fresh, inventory must be transferred to hospitals so that requests are made for an emergency inventory, and a new collection of equipment and shipments can be continuously built for new demands.

The concept is that a group of skilled staff is formed to operate in hospitals for a few weeks each year to maintain their expertise and experience in new equipment to supplement regular hospital personnel in the event of a significant crisis. This will also include trained personnel. While these strategies may seem drastic, global crises such as the COVID-19 19 pandemic already warn of the inadequate conventional procedures. In times of crisis, we are planning for oil and weapons scarcity. The fact that medical supplies are just as essential is now abundantly obvious.

Leave a Better World

Beyond learning about COVID-19, you can also get involved and leave the world better off without being an influential figure. This can be in two ways. Volunteering your service to a nearby clinic or work in a rural area without many doctors and nurses will make a huge difference. Think about making small positive changes to the daily lives of people and improving things.

Advocacy is needed to push our political leaders to take these issues seriously. This can be through lobbying or getting involved with NGOs who are doing advocacy. It can also be through attending talks and writing letters. However, in a sense, making it clear to leadership that these issues are essential and providing support through research.

It also involves thinking that we are global citizens. As people migrate and make friends through social media across the world, we start thinking of each other. We are all in the same boat and not the country or city of birth.

"I mean, this thing is not going away. Even when the virus is gone, the devastation left by people not being able to work for months who were holding on paycheck to paycheck, who have used up their savings – people are going to be in need. So, my thing is, look in your own neighborhood, in your own backyard to see how you can serve and where your service is most essential. That is the real essential work, I think, for people of means."

- Oprah Winfrey

In some ways, that maybe one of the most powerful legacies of COVID-19, MERS, and other infectious outbreaks. If we can change our perspective about each other, then our investment and engagement with global health shall make a difference. It is less about charity but more about solidarity, which is a potentially powerful thing.

Notes

Chapter 1: INTRODUCTION

1. Backer JA, Klinkenberg D, Wallinga J. Incubation period of 2019 novel coronavirus (2019-nCoV) infections among travelers from Wuhan, China, 20-28 January 2020. Euro Surveill. 2020;25(5).
2. Baldwin W. Ventilator manufacturers: we can ramp up production five-fold. Forbes. 14 March 2020. www.forbes.com/sites/baldwin/2020/03/14/ventilator-manufacturers-we-can-ramp-up-production-five-fold/#10246ae65e9a.
3. Balmer C, Pollina E. Italy's Lombardy asks retired health workers to join coronavirus fight. World Economic Forum, Reuters. 2020 (https://www.weforum.org/agenda/2020/03/italys-lombardy-etired-health-workers-coronavirus-covid19-pandemic. opens in new tab).
4. Brooks SK, Webster RK, Smith LE, et al. The psychological impact of quarantine and how to reduce it: a rapid review of the evidence. Lancet 2020; 395:912-920.

5. CDC. How to Protect Yourself. Atlanta, GA; 2020. Available at: https://www.cdc.gov/coronavirus/2019-ncov/prepare/prevention.html. Accessed March 20, 2020.

6. Chopra V, Toner E, Waldhorn R, Washer L. How should U.S. hospitals prepare for coronavirus disease 2019 (COVID-19)? Ann Intern, Med. 2020. [Epub ahead of print March 11, 2020].

7. Doyeon Lee, Yoseob Heo, Keunhwan Kim. (2020) A Strategy for International Cooperation in the COVID-19 Pandemic Era: Focusing on National Scientific Funding Data. Healthcare 8:3, 204.

8. Li JY, You Z, Wang Q, Zhou ZJ, Qiu Y, Luo R, Ge XY. The epidemic of 2019-novel-coronavirus (2019-nCoV) pneumonia and insights for emerging infectious diseases in the future. Microbes Infect. 2020;22(2):80-5.

9. MacIntyre CR. On a knife's edge of a COVID-19 pandemic: is containment still possible? Public Health Res Pract. 2020;30(1):3012000.

10. Meo SA, Alhowikan AM, Al-Khlaiwi T, Meo IM, Halepoto DM, Iqbal M, Usmani AM, Hajjar W, Ahmed N. Novel coronavirus 2019-nCoV: prevalence, biological and clinical characteristics comparison with SARS-CoV and MERS-CoV. Eur Rev Med Pharmacol Sci. 2020;24(4):2012-9.

11. Pfefferbaum B, Schonfeld D, Flynn BW, et al. The H1N1 crisis: a case study of integrating mental and behavioral

health in public health crises. Disaster Med Public Health Prep 2012; 6:67-71.

12. Rishu AH, Marinoff N, Julien L, Dumitrascu M, Marten N, Eggertson S, et al. Time required to initiate outbreak and pandemic observational research. J Crit Care. 2017;40:7–10.

13. Sambala EZ, Manderson L. Anticipation and response: pandemic influenza in Malawi, 2009. Glob Health Action. 2017;10(1):1341225.

14. Stein R. COVID-19 and rationally layered social distancing. Int J Clin Pract. 2020: e13501.

15. WHO. 2020. Report on the WHO-China joint mission on Coronavirus disease 2019 (COVID-19), 16–24 February 2020

Chapter 2: COVID –19 Pandemic

16. Bauchner H, Fontanarosa PB, Livingston EH. Conserving supply of personal protective equipment—a call for ideas. JAMA. 2020; (published online March 20.) DOI:10.1001/jama.2020.4770

17. Card, K. J. et al. UV sterilization of personal protective equipment with idle laboratory biosafety cabinets during the COVID-19 pandemic. https://doi.org/10.1101/2020.03.25.20043489 (2020).

18. Database of Systematic Reviews 2019, Issue 7. Art. No.: CD011621. Disease (COVID -19). March 2020.

19. Ellram, Lisa M., Strategic Cost Management in the Supply Chain: A Purchasing and Supply Management

20. Ericksen, Paul D., and Rajan Suri, "Managing the Extended Enterprise," Purchasing Today, Vol. 12, No. 2, infectious diseases due to exposure to contaminated body fluids in healthcare staff. Cochrane

21. Livingston E, Desai A, Berkwits M. Sourcing personal protective equipment during the COVID-19 pandemic. JAMA. 2020; (published online March 28.) DOI:10.1001/jama.2020.5317

22. Moorman, C., Deshpandé, R., Zaltman, G. (1993). Factors affecting trust in market research relationships. Journal of Marketing, 57(1), 81–101.

23. Patel, A. et al. Personal protective equipment supply chain: lessons learned from recent public health emergency responses. Health Security. 15, 244–252 (2017).

24. Patel, A. et al. Personal protective equipment supply chain: lessons learned from recent public health emergency responses. Health Security. 15, 244–252 (2017).

25. Schniederjans, D.G., Curado, C., & Khalajhedayati, M. (2020). Supply chain digitization trends: An integration of knowledge management. International Journal of Production Economics.

26. Verbeek_JH, Rajamaki_B, Ijaz_S et al. Personal protective equipment for preventing highly

27. World Health Organization. Rational use of personal protective equipment (PPE) for coronavirus

Chapter 3: Personal Protective Equipment (PPE) & Supply Relationship Management (SRM)

28. Bradsher K, Alderman L. The world needs masks. China makes them — but has been hoarding them. New York Times. March 16, 2020 (https://www.nytimes.com/2020/03/13/business/masks-china-coronavirus.html. opens in new tab).

29. Coakley, M. F. et al. The NIH 3D Print Exchange: a public resource for scientific and biomedical 3D prints. 3D Print Addit. Manuf. 1, 137–140 (2014).

30. Curran J. Medical device manufacturing in the U.S. IBISWorld Industry Report 33451b. April 2020. Accessed at https://clients1-ibisworld-com.pitt.idm.oclc.org/reports/us/industry/competitivelandscape.aspx?entid=764.

31. EducationACFGM. ACGME Program Requirements for Graduate Medical Education in Orthopedic Surgery; 2019.

32. Goodnough A. Some hospitals are close to running out of crucial masks for coronavirus. The New York Times. 9 March 2020. Accessed at www.nytimes.com/2020/03/09/health/coronavirus-n95-face-masks.html.

33. Hoehl S, Rabenau H, Berger A, et al. Evidence of SARS-CoV-2 infection in returning travelers from Wuhan, China. N Engl J Med 2020; 382:1278-1280.

34. Hufford A. 3M CEO on N95 masks: 'demand exceeds our production capacity.' The Wall Street Journal. 2 April 2020. Accessed at www.wsj.com/articles/3m-ceo-on-n95-masks-demand-exceeds-our-production-capacity-11585842928.

35. Jacobs A, Richtel M, Baker M. 'At war with no ammo': doctors say shortage of protective gear is dire. New York Times. March 19, 2020 (https://www.nytimes.com/2020/03/19/health/coronavirus-masks-shortage.html. opens in new tab).

36. Ranney ML Griffeth V Jha AK. Critical supply shortages—the need for ventilators and personal protective equipment during the Covid-19 pandemic. N Engl J Med. 2020; 382: e41

Chapter 4: Medical Supplies & Geo-economic   Challenges

37. Carlos del Rio, Preeti N. Malani. COVID-19—New Insights on a Rapidly Changing Epidemic. JAMA. 2020;323(14):1339-1340.

38. Coronavirus Resource Center. COVID-19 map. Baltimore, MD: Johns Hopkins University; 2020. Available from: https://coronavirus.jhu.edu/map.html. Accessed 2020 May 17

39. Fatorachian, H., & Kazemi, H. (2020). A critical investigation of industry in manufacturing: Theoretical operationalization framework. Production Planning & Control, 29 (8),633 -.644

40. FDA Guidance on Conduct of Clinical Trials of Medical Products during COVID-19 Public Health Emergency (https://www.fda.gov/regulatory-information/search-fda-guidance-documents/fda-guidance-conduct-clinical-trials-medical-products-during-covid-19-public-health-emergency).

41. Fink S. Worst-case estimates for U.S. coronavirus deaths. New York Times. March 18, 2020 (https://www.nytimes.com/2020/03/13/us/coronavirus-deaths-estimate.html. opens in new tab).

42. Hobbs, J.E. (2020) Food supply chains during the COVID-19 pandemic, Canadian

43. Jessop ZM, Dobbs TD, Ali SR, Combellack E, Clancy R, Ibrahim N, Jovic TH, Kaur AJ, Nijran A, O'Neill TB, Whitaker IS. Personal Protective Equipment (PPE) for Surgeons during COVID-19 Pandemic: A Systematic Review of Availability, Usage, and Rationing. Br J Surg. 2020 May 12. Journal of Agricultural Economics, https://doi.org/10.1111/cjag.12237

44. Laan E., Dalen J., Rohrmoser M., Simpson R., 2016. Demand forecasting and order Management, 45(1), 114-122.

45. Monczka, Robert M., Robert J. Trent, Robert B. Handfield, Purchasing and Supply Chain Management, 2nd edition, Cincinnati, Ohio: South-Western College Publishing, 2002. planning for humanitarian logistics: An empirical assessment, Journal of Operations

46. Team, IHME COVID-19 health service utilization forecasting, & Murray, C. J. (2020a). Forecasting COVID-19 impact on hospital bed-days, ICU-days, ventilator-days, and deaths by US state in the next 4 months. MedRxiv, 2020.03.27.20043752. doi: 10.1101/2020.03.27.20043752

47. Team, IHME COVID-19 health service utilization forecasting, & Murray, C. J. (2020b). Forecasting the impact of the first wave of the COVID-19 pandemic on hospital demand and deaths for the USA and European Economic Area countries. MedRxiv, 2020.04.21.20074732. doi: 10.1101/2020.04.21.20074732

Chapter 5: Rights of Fulfilment During Pandemics

48. Matt Phillips, "What's gotten into the price of cheese," *The New York Times,* June 22, 2020, https://www.ny-times.com/2020/06/22/business/cheese-cheddar-prices.html.

49. A.M. Campbell. An increasing risk of family violence during the Covid-19 pandemic: Strengthening community

collaborations to save lives.Forensic Science International: Reports (2020), p. 100089

50. S. Funk, E. Gilad, C. Watkins, V.A. Jansen. The spread of awareness and its impact on epidemic outbreaks. Proceedings of the National Academy of Sciences, 106 (16) (2009), pp. 6872-6877

51. B. Jaworski, A.K. Kohli, A. Sahay. Market-driven versus driving markets

52. Jordà, Òscar, Sanjay R. Singh, Alan M. Taylor. 2020. "Longer-Run Economic Consequences of

53. Pandemics," Federal Reserve Bank of San Francisco Working Paper 2020-09. https://doi.org/10.24148/wp2020-09

54. Dee-Ann Durbin, "Where's the beef? Production shutdown leads to shortages" *The Associated Press*, May 7, 2020, https://ap-news.com/1ace47a100d73ce690990d73e597db22.

55. J.T. Cacioppo, L.C. Hawkley. Perceived social isolation and cognition.Trends in Cognitive Sciences, 13 (10) (2009), pp. 447-454

56. Jon Condon and James Nason, "China's coronavirus outbreak will impact beef and cattle trade," *Beef Central,* January 29, 2020, https://www.beefcentral.com/news/chinas-corona-virus-outbreak-will-impact-beef-and-cattle-trade/. Journal of the Academy of Marketing Science, 28 (1) (2000), pp. 45-54

Chapter 6: Re-engineering During Pandemics

57. Al-Shammari A.A.A., Ali H., Al-Ahmad B., Al-Refaei F.H., Al-Sabah S., Jamal M.H. Real-time tracking and forecasting of the COVID-19 outbreak in Kuwait: A mathematical modeling study. MedRxiv. 2020 doi: 10.1101/2020.05.03.20089771. 05.03.20089771.

58. Chen F., Drezner Z., Ryan J.K., Simchi-Levi D. Quantifying the bullwhip effect in a simple supply chain: The impact of forecasting, lead times, and information. Management Science. 2000;46(3):436–443.

59. Gardner E.S., Jr., McKenzie E.D. Forecasting trends in time series. Management Science. 1985;31(10):1237–1246.

60. Govindan K., Mina H., Alavi B. A decision support system for demand management in healthcare supply chains considering the epidemic outbreaks: A case study of coronavirus disease 2019 (COVID-19) Transportation Research Part E: Logistics and Transportation Review. 2020

61. Castro, M.F., .Duarte, J.B., .& Brinca, P. (2020). Measuring sectoral supply and demand shocks during COVID-19. doi: 10.20955/wp.2020.011https://research.stlouisfed.org/wp/more/2020-011

62. Aldrighetti, R., Zennaro, I., Finco, S., & Battini, D. (2019). Healthcare supply chain simulation with disruption

considerations: a case study from Northern Italy. Global Journal of Flexible Systems Management,20, 81–102. https://doi.org/10.1007/s40171-019-00223-8.

63. Paul, S. K., & Chowdhury, P. (2020). A production recovery plan in manufacturing supply chains for a high-demand item during COVID-19. *International Journal of Physical Distribution & Logistics Management*. https://doi.org/10.1108/ijpdlm-04-2020-0127.

64. Salem, M., Van Quaquebeke, N., Besiou, M., & Meyer, L. (2019). Intergroup leadership: How leaders can enhance performance of humanitarian operations. Production and Operations Management,28(11), 2877–2897. https://doi.org/10.1111/poms.13085.

65. Yadav, D. K., & Barve, A. (2016). Modeling post-disaster challenges of humanitarian supply chains: A TISM approach. Global Journal of Flexible Systems Management, 17(3), 321–340.

Chapter 7: Medical Devices Regulation & Harmonization Challenges

66. AMA. CARES Act: AMA COVID-19 pandemic telehealth fact sheet. Available at: https://www.ama-assn.org/delivering-care/public-health/caresact-ama-covid-19-pandemic-telehealth-fact-sheet.

67. American Society of Heating Refrigerating and Air-Conditioning Engineers, American National Standards Institute, American Society for Healthcare Engineering. Ventilation of health care facilities: ASHRAE/ASHE Standard. Atlanta, GA, American Society of Heating, Refrigerating, and Air-Conditioning Engineers, 2008.

68. Asian Development Bank News Release (2020). Developing Asia Growth to Fall in 2020 on COVID-19 Impact. Retrieved from https://www.adb.org/news/developing-asia-growth-fall- 2020-covid-19-impact.

69. CDC. Coronavirus Disease 2019 (COVID-19). Healthcare Facility Guidance. Available at: https://www.cdc.gov/coronavirus/2019-ncov/hcp/guidance-hcf.html.

70. Coakley, M. F. et al. The NIH 3D Print Exchange: a public resource for bioscientific and biomedical 3D prints. 3D Print Addit. Manuf. 1, 137–140 (2014).

71. Green-McKenzie J, Gershon RR, Karkashian C. Infection control practices among correctional healthcare workers: effect of management attitudes and availability of protective equipment and engineering controls. Infection Control and Hospital Epidemiology, 2001, 22(9):555–559 (http://www.ncbi.nlm.nih.gov/entrez/query.fcgi?cmd=Retrieve&db=PubMed&dopt=Citation&list_uids =11732784).

72. Jamieson D.J., Steinberg J.P., Martinello R.A., Perl T.M., Rasmussen S.A. Obstetricians on the coronavirus disease 2019 (COVID-19) front lines and the confusing world of personal protective equipment. Obstet Gynecol. 2020;135:1257–1263.

73. World Health Organization. Rolling updates on coronavirus disease (COVID-19). Available at: https://www.who.int/emergencies/diseases/novel-coronavirus-2019/events-as-they-happen

74. Wosik J, Fudim M, Cameron B, et al. Telehealth transformation: COVID-19 and the rise of virtual care. J Am Med Inform Assoc 2020;27: 957–62.

Chapter 8: Integrating Pandemic Management

75. Agence Nationale de Securité de Médicament et des Produits de Santé [France]. Covid 19 – Ongoing clinical trials. https://www.ansm.sante.fr/Activites/Essais-cliniques/COVID-19-Ongoing-clinical-trials/(offset)/1#paragraph_172505. Published 20 March 2020; last updated 20 May 2020. Accessed 7 July 2020.

76. Agencia Espanola de Medicamentos y Productos Sanitarios [Spain]. Exceptional measures applicable to clinical trials to manage problems arising from the COVID-19 emergency. https://www.aemps.gob.es/informa-en/exceptional-measures-applicable-to-clinical-trials-to-manage-problems-arising-from-the-covid-19-

emergency/?lang=en. Last updated 1 July 2020. Accessed 7 July 2020.

77. European Medicines Agency. ICH E6 (R2) Good clinical practice. https://www.ema.europa.eu/en/ich-e6-r2-good-clinical-practice. Last updated 15 December 2016. Accessed 10 July 2020.

78. McKinsey & Co. COVID-19 implications for life sciences R&D: Recovery and the next normal. https://www.mckinsey.com/industries/pharmaceuticals-and-medical-products/our-insights/covid-19-implications-for-life-sciences-r-and-d-recovery-and-the-next-normal. Published 13 May 2020. Accessed 7 July 2020.

79. Ministry of Health and Regulatory Affairs [UK]. Managing clinical trials during coronavirus (COVID-19): How investigators and sponsors should manage clinical trials during COVID-19. https://www.gov.uk/guidance/managing-clinical-trials-during-coronavirus-covid-19 . Published 19 March 2020; last updated 21 May 2020. Accessed 7 July 2020.

80. OECD (2016), International Regulatory Co-operation: The Role of International Organisations in Fostering Better Rules of Globalisation, OECD Publishing, Paris, https://doi.org/10.1787/9789264244047-en.

81. Paul-Ehrlich Institut [Germany]. Clinical trials during the COVID-19 pandemic. https://www.pei.de/EN/regulation/clinical-trials/covid-19/covid-19-node.html;jsessionid=EF8CC6462B2B1D95828041A7BC8EE810.2_cid319. Updated 26 May 2020. Accessed 7 July 2020.

82. This is documented in a forthcoming work of the OECD Regulatory Policy Division, dedicated to international regulatory co-operation. www.who.int/gho/publications/world_health_statistics/en/.

83. US Food and Drug Administration. Clinical Trials Guidance Documents. https://www.fda.gov/regulatory-information/search-fda-guidance-documents/clinical-trials-guidance-documents. Last updated 21 January 2020. Accessed 10 July 2020.

84. US Food and Drug Administration. FDA guidance on conduct of clinical trials of medical products during COVID-19 public health emergency: Guidance for industry, investigators, and institutional review boards. https://www.fda.gov/media/136238/download. Published March 2020; last updated 2 July 2020. Accessed 7 July 2020.

Chapter 9: Demand Management Style

85. José Guimón, Rajneesh Narula. (2020) Ending the COVID-19 Pandemic Requires More International Collaboration. Research-Technology Management 63:5, 38-41.

86. Centers for Disease Control and Prevention, Coronavirus Disease 2019 (COVID-19): Therapeutic Options (2020), https://www.cdc.gov/coronavirus/2019-ncov/hcp/therapeutic-options.html.

87. FDA, Remdesivir Emergency Use Authorization Letter (2020), https://www.fda.gov/media/137564/download.

88. Gates B. Innovation for pandemics. N Engl J Med 2018; 378:2057-2060.

89. Gates B. The next epidemic — lessons from Ebola. N Engl J Med 2015; 372:1381-4. DOI: 10.1056/NEJMp1502918

90. Koh D. Occupational risks for COVID-19 infection. Occup Med (Lond). 2020;70(1):3-5.

91. Koonin, L. M. (2020). Novel coronavirus disease (COVID-19) outbreak: Now is the time to refresh pandemic plans. Journal of Business Continuity & Emergency Planning,13(4), 1–15.

92. Sambala EZ, Manderson L. Anticipation and response: pandemic influenza in Malawi, 2009. Glob Health Action. 2017;10(1):1341225.

Chapter 10: Hospital Capacity Management

93. Fan, V.Y., Jamison, D.T. and Summers, L.H., 2018. Pandemic risk: how large are the expected losses? Bulletin of the World Health Organization, 96(2), p.129.

94. Gates, B., 2018. Innovation for pandemics. New England Journal of Medicine, 378(22), pp.2057-2060.

95. Li L. China's manufacturing locus in 2025: With a comparison of "made-in-China 2025" and "industry 4.0" Technological Forecasting and Social Change. 2018; 135:66–74.

96. Lin C. Harvard Business Review. 2020. Delivery technology is keeping Chinese cities afloat through coronavirus. https://hbr.org/2020/03/delivery-technology-is-keeping-chinese-cities-afloat-through-coronavirus retrieved on 25 March 2020.

97. Lorenzoni, L., Marino, A., Morgan, D. and James, C., 2019. Health Spending Projections to 2030: New results based on a revised OECD methodology.

98. Schütte, S., Acevedo, P.N.M. and Flahault, A., 2018. Health systems around the world–a comparison of existing health system rankings. Journal of global health, 8(1).

99. Servick K. Cellphone tracking could help stem the spread of coronavirus. Is privacy the price? Science. 2020 doi: 10.1126/science. abb8296.

100. The Lancet COVID-19: Fighting panic with information. The Lancet. 2020; 395:537.

101. Tremlett G. How did Spain get its Coronavirus response so wrong? 2020. https://www.theguardian.com/world/2020/mar/26/spain-coronavirus-response-analysis

102. Wakefield J. Coronavirus: Tracking app aims for one million downloads. 2020. https://www.bbc.co.uk/news/technology-52033210

103. Westcott B. China has made eating wild animals illegal after the coronavirus outbreak. But ending the trade wont' be easy. 2020. https://edition.cnn.com/2020/03/05/asia/china-coronavirus-wildlife-consumption-ban-intl-hnk/index.html/

104. WHO Global surveillance for COVID-19 disease caused by human infection with novel coronavirus (COVID-19) 2020. https://www.who.int/publications-detail/global-surveillance-for-human-infection-with-novel-coronavirus-(2019-ncov)/ accessed 9 March 2020.

105. Hohenstein, N-O., Feisel, E., Hartmann, E., Giunipero, L., 2015. Research on the phenomenon of supply chain resilience A systematic review and paths for further investigation, International Journal of Physical Distribution & Logistics Management,45(1/2), 90 – 117

106. Hübner, A., Wollenburg, J., Holzapfel, A., 2016. Retail logistics in the transition from multi-channel to Omni-channel, International Journal of Physical Distribution &Logistics Management, 46(6/7), 562 – 583

107. Melacini, M., Perotti, S., Rasini, M., Tappia, E., 2018. E-fulfillment and distribution in Omni-channel retailing: a systematic literature review, International Journal of Physical Distribution & Logistics Management, 48(4), 391-414

108. The World Health Organization (WHO). Situation report - 18. Feb 7, 2020. [EB/OL]

109. https://www.who.int/docs/default-source/coronaviruse/transcripts/transcriptcoronavirus-press-conference-full07feb2020-_nal.pdf?sfvrsn=3beba1c0_2

110. We are using cookies to give you the best experience on our website, but you are free to manage these at any time. To continue with our standard settings, click "Accept". To find out more and manage your cookies, click "Manage cookies"15/07/2020 Supply Chain and Technology Innovation during COVID-19 Outbreak | Emerald Publishinghttps://www.emeraldgrouppublishing.com/journal/ijpdlm/supply-chain-and-technology-innovation-during-covid-19-outbreak 6/6

111. Wieland, A., Wallenburg, C.M., 2013. The influence of relational competencies on supply chain resilience: a relational view, International Journal of Physical Distribution & Logistics Management, 43(4), 300-320,https://doi.org/10.1108/IJPDLM-08-2012-0243

112. Dasaklis TK., Costas PP., Nikolaos PR., 2012. Epidemics control and logistics operations: A review, International Journal of Production Economics, 139: 393-410.

113. Gupta S., Martin KS., Reza ZF., Niki M., 2016. Disaster management from a POM perspective: Mapping a new domain, Production and Operations Management,25(10): 1611-1637.

114. Wollenburg, J., Hübner, A., Kuhn, H., Trautrims, A., 2018. From bricks-and-mortar to bricks-and-clicks: Logistics networks in omni-channel grocery retailing, International Journal of Physical Distribution & Logistics Management, https://doi.org/10.1108/IJPDLM-10-2016-0290

Chapter 11. Reimagining Healthcare for Pandemics

115. Hohenstein, N-O., Feisel, E., Hartmann, E., Giunipero, L., 2015. Research on the phenomenon of supply chain resilience A systematic review and paths for further

116. Investigation, International Journal of Physical Distribution & Logistics Management, 45(1/2), 90 – 117

117. Hübner, A., Wollenburg, J., Holzapfel, A., 2016. Retail logistics in the transition from multi-channel to omni-channel, International Journal of Physical Distribution & Logistics Management, 46(6/7), 562 - 583

118. Melacini, M., Perotti, S., Rasini, M., Tappia, E., 2018. E-ful-fillment and distribution in omni-channel retailing: a systematic literature review, International Journal of

119. Physical Distribution & Logistics Management, 48(4), 391-414

120. The World Health Organization (WHO). Situation report - 18. Feb 7, 2020. [EB/OL]

121. https://www.who.int/docs/default-source/coronaviruse/transcripts/transcriptcoronavirus-press-conference-full07feb2020-_nal.pdf?sfvrsn=3beba1c0_2

122. 15/07/2020 Supply Chain and Technology Innovation during COVID-19 Outbreak | Emerald Publishing

123. https://www.emeraldgrouppublishing.com/journal/ijpdlm/supply-chain-and-technology-innovation-during-covid-19-outbreak 6/6

124. Wieland, A., Wallenburg, C.M., 2013. The infuence of relational competencies on supply chain resilience: a relational view, International Journal of Physical Distribution & Logistics Management, 43(4), 300-320, https://doi.org/10.1108/IJPDLM-08-2012-0243

Chapter 12. Conclusions

125. Dasaklis TK., Costas PP., Nikolaos PR., 2012. Epidemics control and logistics operations: A review, International Journal of Production Economics, 139: 393-410.

126. Gupta S., Martin KS., Reza ZF., Niki M., 2016. Disaster management from a POM perspective: Mapping a new domain, Production and Operations Management, 25(10): 1611-1637.

127. Wollenburg, J., Hübner, A., Kuhn, H., Trautrims, A., 2018. From bricks-and-mortar to

128. Bricks-and-clicks: Logistics networks in omni-channel grocery retailing, International Journal of Physical Distribution & Logistics Management, https://doi.org/10.1108/IJPDLM-10-2016-0290

Author's Biography

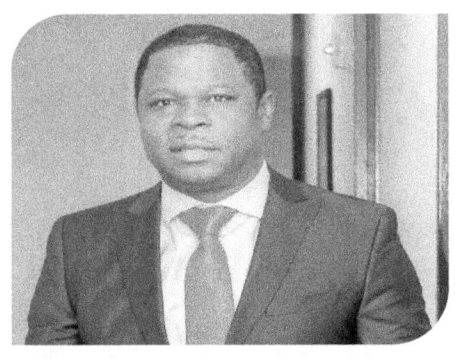

Dr. Ebot Eyong is the Founder and CEO of E & E Medicals and Consulting. A full-service engineering, regulatory, and sales corporation for advanced medical devices. Dr. Eyong is a Biomedical Engineer, Quality Assurance, and Regulatory Consultant. For more than a decade, he has dedicated his career to helping global medical device companies and regulatory agencies find success in the healthcare industry. He is also a strong advocate for harmonizing medical device regulations around the globe.

During the Ebola outbreak, as the President of the Orphan Kids Help Foundation (OKHF), he worked with international organizations to help support kids in the sub-Saharan region of Africa who were affected by the virus. Dr. Eyong worked with healthcare experts and Epidemiologists, shedding light on the problems posed by epidemics and the consequences of the lack of medical supplies in that region. Dr. Eyong earned his doctorate in Engineering Management from Walden University.